VEGAN DIET COOKBOOK FOR
VESTIBULAR MIGRAINE

Wholesome Dishes for Headache Management"

Anita F. MS RDN McCluskey

TABLE OF CONTENTS

INTRODUCTION

Welcome to the "Vegan Diet Cookbook for Vestibular Migraines" by Anita F. Mccluskey. This book is a helpful guide for people dealing with vestibular migraines. These migraines cause vertigo and other tough symptoms that affect daily life. Anita F. Mccluskey understands how important food is in managing these symptoms. That's why she created this cookbook full of tasty vegan recipes.

This cookbook not only shows the health benefits of plant-based eating but also helps you make meals that are good for migraines and delicious. Whether you're new to vegan food or looking for new ideas, each recipe is designed to make you feel good and meet the dietary needs linked to vestibular migraines.

Inside, you'll find a range of recipes from energizing breakfasts to comforting dinners and sweet desserts. Each recipe is made carefully to avoid common migraine triggers and give you lots of nutrition and flavor. Anita F. Mccluskey's experience as a chef and her understanding of vestibular migraines mean every dish in this book supports your health and tastes great.

Let this cookbook be your guide to better health and tasty meals with the "Vegan Diet Cookbook for Vestibular Migraines." Whether you want relief from symptoms, a balanced vegan diet, or just delicious food, this book has what you need to feel your best.

Chapter 1: Understanding Vestibular Migraine

Vestibular migraine is a complex type of headache that affects the brain and balance systems. This chapter explains how these two systems interact. It covers symptoms, how doctors diagnose it, and the reasons behind why it happens. The goal is to help readers understand how vestibular migraine affects daily life and how to manage it effectively.

1.1 What is Vestibular Migraine?

Vestibular migraine is a type of migraine that involves episodes of vertigo or dizziness as a significant symptom, along with typical migraine symptoms such as headache, sensitivity to light and sound, and nausea. It is considered a neurological disorder where the vestibular system, which contributes to balance and spatial orientation, is affected during migraine attacks. People with vestibular migraine may experience vertigo or a sensation of spinning or swaying, often accompanied by head pain or discomfort. These episodes can vary in frequency and intensity from person to person. Management typically involves a combination of lifestyle changes, medication, and sometimes vestibular rehabilitation therapy.

1.2 Symptoms and Triggers

- **Dizziness:** Feeling like things are spinning or being off-balance.
- **Migraine Symptoms:** Headaches (often throbbing and on one side), sensitivity to light and sound, nausea, and sometimes vomiting.
- **Vision Problems:** Blurred vision or seeing flashes of light.

<u>*Triggers*</u>

Vestibular migraines can be triggered by various factors:

Stress or Anxiety

- <u>**Hormonal Changes:**</u> Such as during periods of menopause.

- <u>**Things in the Environment:**</u> Bright lights, loud noises, or strong smells.

- <u>**Physical Factors:**</u> Being tired, not sleeping enough, or doing too much physical activity.

- <u>**Certain Foods or Drinks:**</u> Like coffee, alcohol, or processed foods.

- <u>**Weather Changes:**</u> Such as changes in air pressure.

- **_Medications:_** Some medicines can bring on migraines.

Diagnosis

Doctors diagnose vestibular migraine by asking about your health history, doing a physical exam, and sometimes doing tests like balance tests or scans to rule out other causes.

Treatment

Managing vestibular migraines usually involves:

1. **Medicine:** Pain relievers, drugs to stop nausea, or regular medicines to prevent migraines.

2. **Lifestyle Changes:** Learning to manage stress, keeping a regular sleep schedule, and changing your diet.

3.Physical Therapy: Exercises to improve balance and make you less sensitive to motion.

4.Alternative Therapies: Things like acupuncture or counseling to reduce stress.

Outlook

While vestibular migraines can be hard to handle, many people get relief with the right treatment and lifestyle changes. Working closely with your doctor to find out what triggers your migraines and making a plan to treat them can help.

Conclusion

Vestibular migraine is a complex condition that mixes migraine symptoms with problems in balance. Knowing the signs, what sets it off, and how to treat it is key for people affected by this condition to manage symptoms and live better.

Chapter 2: The Vegan Diet and Vestibular Health

This chapter looks at how vegan diets affect balance and the vestibular system, which helps with spatial awareness. It covers what nutrients are important, the good things about vegan diets for balance, and the challenges. The chapter explains how going vegan can affect the inner ear and help keep balance healthy.

2.1 Benefits of a Vegan Diet for Migraine Management

A vegan diet excludes all animal products like meat, dairy, and eggs, and it offers several health benefits that can help manage migraines and support overall vestibular health.

1.Less Inflammation: Vegan diets are rich in anti-inflammatory foods such as fruits, vegetables, whole grains, nuts, and seeds. Chronic inflammation is linked to health issues including migraines. By reducing inflammation, vegan diets may lessen how often and how severe migraines are.

2. _Better Gut Health:_ The gut plays a big role in immune function and inflammation. Vegan diets, which are high in fiber and plant-based foods, support a diverse microbiome that can improve overall health, including managing migraines.

3. _Reduced Triggers:_ Some foods like processed meats, aged cheeses, and alcohol can trigger migraines for some people. A vegan diet naturally avoids these triggers, potentially lowering the chances of migraine attacks.

4. _Balanced Nutrition:_ A well-planned vegan diet provides essential nutrients like vitamins C, E, and magnesium, which are important for brain health and reducing migraine symptoms.

2.2 Nutritional Tips

While a vegan diet has many health benefits, it's important to ensure you get the right nutrition to support vestibular health and well-being.

1.Protein: Get protein from plant sources like beans, lentils, tofu, tempeh, quinoa, and nuts. Mixing different plant proteins throughout the day ensures you get all the amino acids your body needs.

2.Vitamins and Minerals: Pay attention to getting enough vitamin B12, vitamin D, iron, calcium, zinc, and omega-3 fatty acids. Vegans may need supplements for vitamin B12 and possibly vitamin D since these nutrients are mainly found in animal products.

3.Omega-3 Fats: Sources like flaxseeds, chia seeds, walnuts, and algae supplements provide essential omega-3 fatty acids that are good for brain health and reducing inflammation.

4.Calcium: Get calcium from fortified plant milks, tofu, leafy greens (such as kale and collard greens), and almonds to support bone health and nerve function.

5. Iron: Plant sources of iron include lentils, chickpeas, beans, spinach, and fortified cereals. Eating foods rich in vitamin C (like citrus fruits and bell peppers) with iron-rich foods helps your body absorb iron better.

6. Meal Planning: Plan your meals to include a variety of foods to ensure you get all the nutrients you need. Consulting a registered dietitian or healthcare provider can give you personalized advice to make sure your diet is healthy and balanced.

In conclusion, adopting a vegan diet can potentially help manage migraines and improve overall vestibular health due to its anti-inflammatory properties and nutrient-rich foods. Make sure to plan your diet carefully to meet your nutritional needs and enjoy better health and quality of life.

Chapter 3: Breakfast Recipes

Chapter 3 of this cookbook focuses on breakfast recipes. It's filled with tasty and nutritious dishes that will wake you up and give you energy in the morning. You'll find traditional favorites like pancakes and scrambled eggs, as well as creative meals like breakfast bowls and pastries. Whether you need something quick for weekdays or a leisurely brunch idea for weekends, these recipes will help you start your day with delicious food.

3.1 Energizing breakfast

1.Vegan Breakfast Bowl with Low Carbs and Superfoods

Enjoy a colorful vegan breakfast bowl filled with nutritious ingredients to kickstart your day. Packed with superfoods like creamy avocado, seasoned tofu, fresh cherry tomatoes, and chia seeds, all topped with a tangy lemon tahini dressing. It's a tasty and healthy way to begin your morning!

This filling breakfast is perfect for vegan keto diets because it's low in carbs, high in protein and healthy fats, and has very little sugar. It keeps you satisfied and energized from morning to early afternoon.

<u>Preparation time</u>

- Prep: 5 mins
- Total Time: 5 mins
- Servings: 1
- Calories: 500 kcal

<u>Ingredients:</u>

- 1 cup unsweetened almond milk (or any non-dairy milk)
- 1/4 cup vegan protein powder
- 2 tbsp chia seeds

- 1/2 tbsp hemp seeds
- 2 tbsp unsweetened coconut flakes
- Optional Mix-ins: mixed berries, chopped pecans, chopped walnuts

Instructions:

1. Mix almond milk, protein powder, chia seeds, hemp seeds, and coconut flakes in a jar.
2. Shake well to blend the ingredients thoroughly.
3. Chill overnight in the fridge.
4. In the morning, add mixed berries and nuts.
5. Enjoy the cold!

Notes:

- Start with 3/4 cup almond milk for a thicker consistency.
- Adjust sweetness based on your protein powder choice.

- For no protein powder, use less almond milk and increase dry ingredients slightly.

This easy and healthy breakfast bowl is ideal for vegans, gluten-free diets, and potentially keto-friendly lifestyles.

Nutrition information:

This meal contains:
- 500 calories
- 20 grams of carbohydrates
- 30 grams of protein
- 35 grams of fat (8 grams of which are saturated)
- 521 milligrams of sodium
- 237 milligrams of potassium
- 12 grams of fiber
- 4 grams of sugar
- 403 milligrams of calcium
- 8.9 milligrams of iron

2.Vegan Buckwheat Pancakes

These vegan buckwheat pancakes are a tasty twist on a traditional breakfast favorite. They're made with healthy ingredients like buckwheat flour, almond milk, and flaxseed meal, giving you a wholesome start to your day. Sweetened with maple syrup and flavored with vanilla, each bite is satisfying and comforting. You can top them with fresh berries, coconut yogurt, or chopped nuts for a delicious and nutritious morning treat that everyone will love, whether they're vegan or not.

Preparation time

- Prep: 10 mins
- Cook: 10 mins
- Total: 20 mins
- Servings: 3
- caloriesHelps: 269

Ingredients:

- 1/2 cup buckwheat flour
- 1/2 cup brown rice flour
- 2 tsp baking powder
- 1/2 tsp cinnamon
- Pinch of salt
- 1/4 cup unsweetened applesauce
- 1 tbsp melted coconut oil or butter
- 1 tsp vanilla extract
- 1 tsp white vinegar
- 1 cup non-dairy milk

Instructions:

1. Mix buckwheat flour, brown rice flour, baking powder, cinnamon, and salt in a bowl.
2. Create a well in the center; add applesauce, melted coconut oil, vanilla extract, vinegar, and non-dairy milk.
3. Stir until smooth; let batter rest for 5 minutes.
4. Heat a non-stick skillet over medium heat; lightly grease.

5. Pour 1/4 cup batter per pancake onto the skillet.

6. Cook until bubbles form, about 2-3 minutes per side.

7. Serve warm with toppings like maple syrup or fresh fruit.

Notes:

- Makes about 6 pancakes.
- Add 1 tsp sugar if using unsweetened applesauce.
- Substitute all-purpose flour for a different texture.

Nutrition (per serving, 2 pancakes):

- Calories: 269 kcal
- Carbs: 42 g
- Protein: 10 g
- Fat: 9 g
- Saturated Fat: 6 g
- Sodium: 42 mg
- Fiber: 4 g

- Sugars: 5 g
- Vitamins: A (139 IU), C (1 mg)
- Minerals: Calcium (223 mg), Iron (2 mg)

3. Vegan Banana Bread Waffles

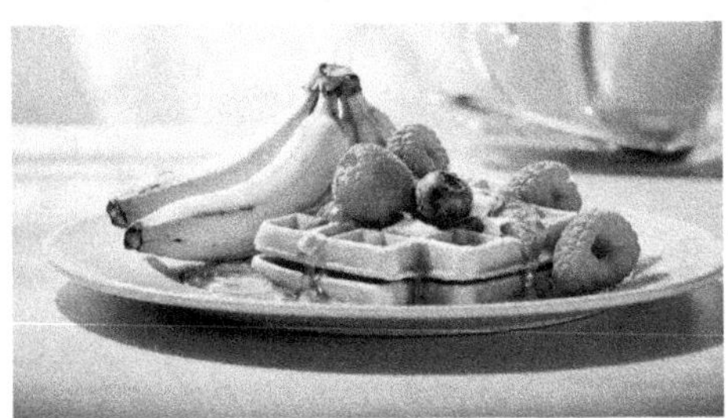

"Enjoy our Vegan Banana Bread Waffles, a tasty blend of banana bread and fluffy waffles. Each bite is crispy outside and soft inside, with a delicious banana flavor. They're made with almond milk, whole wheat flour, and a hint of cinnamon, and they're vegan and nutritious. Eat them warm with maple syrup or dairy-free yogurt for a wholesome and satisfying breakfast treat."

These Vegan Banana Bread Waffles have a lovely golden-brown color with crispy outsides and soft insides filled with crunchy walnuts. They're quick to make in less than 15 minutes, perfect for a relaxed morning treat. Made without dairy or eggs and naturally sweetened, they're a guilt-free indulgence. Enjoy them as a healthy breakfast choice for vegans, offering a delicious mix of flavors and textures that satisfy cravings while being mindful of health.

To make banana bread waffles, you'll need:

Ingredients:
1. Flour (all-purpose, spelt, or whole-wheat)
2. Baking powder (to help the batter rise)
3. Pinch of sea salt (balances sweetness)
4. Optional ground cinnamon (for a warm flavor)
5. Overripe bananas (with brown spots for sweetness; thaw if frozen)
6. Maple syrup (for natural sweetness)
7. Sunflower oil (or canola/olive oil)
8. Unsweetened almond milk (or oat, soy, or cashew milk at room temperature)

9. Apple cider vinegar (or lemon juice)
10. Walnuts (chopped, or chocolate chips)

Tools:

- Medium bowl
- Whisk
- Large bowl
- Fork or potato masher
- Silicon spatula
- Waffle iron (non-stick)

Follow these steps and use these tools to make delicious banana bread waffles.

Preparation time

- Preparation: 5 minutes
- Cooking: 10 minutes
- Total: 15 minutes
- Course: Breakfast, Brunch, Dessert
- Diet: Vegan
- Yield: Makes 4 waffles
- Calories: 326 per serving

- 140g all-purpose flour
- 2 tbsp baking powder
- Pinch of sea salt
- Optional: ¼ tsp ground cinnamon
- 200g ripe bananas (about 2 small bananas)
- 2 tbsp maple syrup
- 2 tbsp sunflower oil (or canola oil)
- 5 tbsp unsweetened almond milk (or any plant-based milk)
- 1 tbsp apple cider vinegar (or lemon juice)
- 40g chopped walnuts (about ¼ cup)
- Baking spray (if your waffle iron isn't non-stick)

Optional Toppings:

- Sliced banana
- Chopped walnuts
- Maple syrup

Instructions:

1. In a medium bowl, mix together flour, baking powder, sea salt, and cinnamon (if using). Set aside.

2. In a large bowl, mash bananas until smooth. Add maple syrup, sunflower oil, almond milk, and apple cider vinegar. Mix well.

3. Gradually add the flour mixture to the banana mixture, stirring until smooth. Fold in chopped walnuts.

4. Preheat your waffle iron and spray with baking spray if necessary. Pour batter onto the iron, close, and cook until golden brown (about 7-10 minutes per waffle). Repeat with remaining batter.

5. Serve warm waffles topped with sliced banana, chopped walnuts, and maple syrup if desired.

- For a healthier option, use spelt or whole-wheat flour instead of all-purpose flour.
- Substitute walnuts with other nuts or chocolate chips if preferred.

- Freeze waffles in a zip-lock bag or airtight container for up to 3 months. Reheat in a 175°C (350°F) oven for 5-10 minutes or microwave for 1 minute.

Nutrition Facts (per waffle):

- Calories: 326 kcal
- Total Fat: 14.1 g
- Saturated Fat: 1.4 g
- Cholesterol: 0 mg
- Total Carbohydrate: 46.2 g
- Fiber: 3.1 g
- Sugar: 12.4 g
- Protein: 5.8 g

- Sodium: 49 mg
- Potassium: 284 mg
- Iron: 2.1 mg

4.Vegan Blueberry Muffin

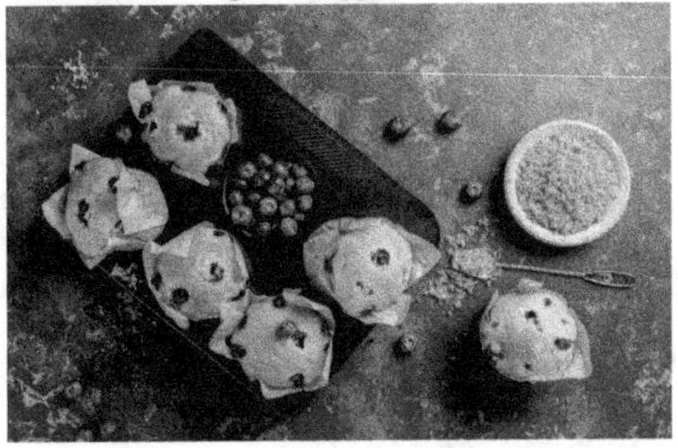

Vegan Blueberry Muffins are deliciously fluffy with juicy blueberries in every bite. They're made without any animal products, perfect for plant-based diets. Each moist muffin is naturally sweetened by blueberries, pleasing vegans and non-vegans alike. Enjoy them for breakfast, a snack, or with a warm drink—they're a wholesome and guilt-free treat.

Here's an easy and delicious vegan blueberry muffin recipe that's better than what you find in bakeries! They're super fluffy and moist, made with just 7 basic ingredients in one bowl.

Preparation time
- Prep Time: 15 minutes
- Cook Time: 25 minutes
- Total Time: 40 minutes
- Servings: 12 muffins

Ingredients:
- Dry Ingredients:
- 2 ⅓ cups (290g) all-purpose flour (use gluten-free if needed)
- ¾ cup (150g) granulated sugar (light brown or coconut sugar can also be used)
- 3 teaspoons baking powder
- 2 teaspoons lemon zest (optional)
- ½ teaspoon ground cinnamon (optional)
- Pinch of salt

<u>*Wet Ingredients:*</u>

- 1 cup (250g) room temperature dairy-free milk
- ½ cup (125g) neutral-flavored oil
- 1 tablespoon apple cider vinegar (optional)
- 1 teaspoon vanilla extract
- 1 ¾ cups (260g) fresh or frozen blueberries (don't thaw if using frozen)

<u>*Optional Topping:*</u>

- 2 tablespoons raw demerara sugar

<u>*Instructions*</u>

1. Preheat your oven to 180°C (350°F) and line a muffin tray with liners.

2. In a large bowl, mix together all the dry ingredients until smooth. Add the wet ingredients (except the blueberries) and stir until

just combined. Fold most of the blueberries into the batter, saving some for topping.

3. Use a scoop or spoon to fill the muffin liners evenly.

4. Optionally, sprinkle the remaining blueberries and raw demerara sugar on top of each muffin.

5. Bake at 180°C (350°F) for about 25 minutes if using fresh blueberries, or 30 minutes if using frozen. To check if they're done, insert a toothpick into the center; it should come out clean or with a few crumbs.

6. Let the muffins cool in the tray for 10 minutes, then transfer them to a wire rack to cool completely. Optionally, sprinkle more demerara sugar on top before serving.

7. Enjoy the muffins warm with vegan butter, or let them cool to room temperature. Store

leftovers in an airtight container at room temperature for up to 2 days, in the fridge for 3 days, or freeze for up to 1 month. Note that the sugar topping may soften after the first day.

Note

To measure flour accurately, fluff it up in its container and use a spoon to gently fill a measuring cup, leveling it with a knife. Avoid packing flour into the cup directly from the container to prevent dry and dense muffins. Alternatively, use gram measurements for precise amounts.

For gluten-free vegan blueberry muffins, use 1 ½ cups (150g) almond meal and 1 cup (160g) gluten-free all-purpose flour instead of regular flour.

For vegan lemon blueberry muffins, swap ¼ cup of dairy-free milk with ¼ cup (60g) lemon juice and add 1 tablespoon of lemon zest. These muffins may be denser and have less of a domed top compared to regular blueberry muffins.

You can use melted coconut oil (at room temperature) in the recipe, but be aware it might solidify in cooler temperatures, potentially making the muffins drier. Warm them before serving if needed.

This recipe makes either 12 large muffins or about 6 jumbo café-sized ones.

To bake jumbo muffins, bake them for 25-35 minutes (adjust based on your muffin tin size) or until a skewer comes out clean when inserted.

<u>**Nutritional Information (per serving, without sugar topping):**</u>

- Calories: 246
- Carbohydrates: 35g
- Protein: 3g
- Fat: 11g
- Sodium: 134mg
- Potassium: 46mg
- Fiber: 1g
- Sugar: 15g
- Vitamins: A: 12IU, C: 3mg
- Minerals: Calcium: 91mg, Iron: 1mg

4. Vegan Breakfast Burritos

Vegan breakfast burritos are a tasty morning choice full of plant-based ingredients. They usually include tofu scramble, seasoned black beans, and sautéed veggies like bell peppers and onions, all wrapped in a warm tortilla. Top them with fresh avocado, salsa, and dairy-free cheese or cashew sauce for a delicious and nutritious start to your day!

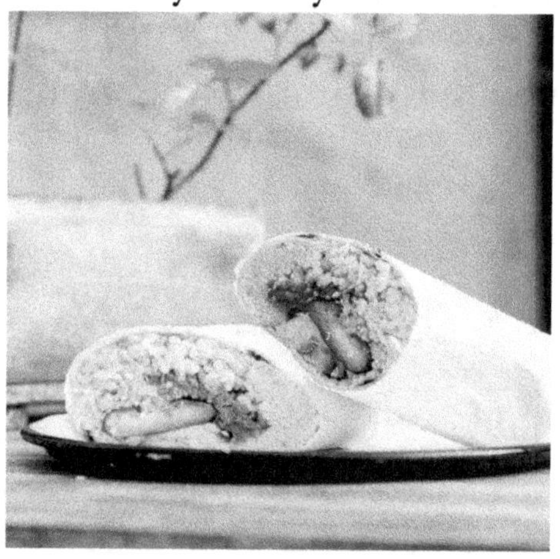

Preparation time

- Preparation time:
- 20 minutes
- Cooking time:
- 30 minutes
- Total time:
- 50 minutes
- Servings:
- 8 burritos

Ingredients

Cheesy Cashew Sauce:

- Start by using 1 1/2 cups of raw cashews.
- Include 3/4 cup of chunky salsa for added flavor.
- Incorporate 1/4 cup of pickled jalapeños.
- Mix in 1/4 cup of the tangy juice from the jalapeño jar.
- Add 1/4 cup of nutritional yeast.
- Season with 1/2 teaspoon of salt to taste.

Hash Adventure:

- Heat 2 tablespoons of olive oil in a pan.
- Add 2 medium russet potatoes, peeled and diced.
- Include 2 medium sweet potatoes, peeled and diced.
- Season with 1 teaspoon of salt and 1/2 teaspoon of black pepper.
- Stir in 1 diced medium red bell pepper.
- Sauté 3 large minced garlic cloves.
- Mix in drained and rinsed pinto beans from a 15-ounce can.

Tofu Tango:

- Heat 1 tablespoon of olive oil in a skillet.
- Crumble a 14.5-ounce block of extra-firm tofu into the pan.
- Sprinkle 2 tablespoons of nutritional yeast.

- Season with 1/2 teaspoon of black salt (or regular salt) and 1/4 teaspoon of turmeric.

The Assembly:

- Warm 8 large tortillas.
- Serve with optional hot sauce, avocado, pico de gallo, and fresh cilantro.

Instructions:

Make the queso:

1. Boil 3-4 cups of water. Pour it over the cashews and let them soak for 5 minutes to 1 hour.

2. Drain the cashews and put them in a blender. Add salsa, jalapeños with their juices, nutritional yeast, and salt. Blend until smooth. Set aside.

Cook the hash:

1. Heat oil in a large skillet over medium heat. Add potatoes, season with salt and pepper, and cover. Cook for 10 minutes.

2. Remove the lid, turn the heat to medium-high, and add red bell pepper. Cook for about 15 minutes, stirring occasionally, until potatoes are golden.

3. Lower the heat to medium, add garlic, and cook for 1-2 minutes. Stir in beans and remove from heat.

Prepare the tofu scramble:

1. Heat olive oil in a skillet over medium heat. Crumble tofu into the pan and cook for 3-4 minutes, stirring often.

2. Add nutritional yeast, black salt, and turmeric. Stir and cook for 5-10 more minutes. Remove from heat.

3. Mix the queso into the tofu scramble.

Assemble the burritos:

1. Place a tortilla flat. Add tofu scramble with queso, then the hash.

2. Optional: Add hot sauce, cilantro, tomatoes, or other toppings. Avoid extra toppings if freezing.

3. Fold the sides of the tortilla over the filling and roll it up.

4. For a crispy burrito, heat oil in a pan and cook each side for about 3 minutes until golden brown.

Serve right away or wrap in foil for freezing. To reheat, warm in a 350°F oven for 20-30 minutes or microwave for 2-3 minutes, flipping halfway through.

Notes:

- For a gluten-free option, use gluten-free tortillas.
- To reduce sodium, use salt-free beans and less salt in the recipes.
- For a soy-free version, use scrambled JUST Egg or chickpea scramble instead of tofu.

- Calories: 476
- Carbs: 57g
- Protein: 18g
- Fat: 21g
- Saturated Fat: 4g
- Sodium: 1115mg
- Fiber: 9g

5. Millet Porridge

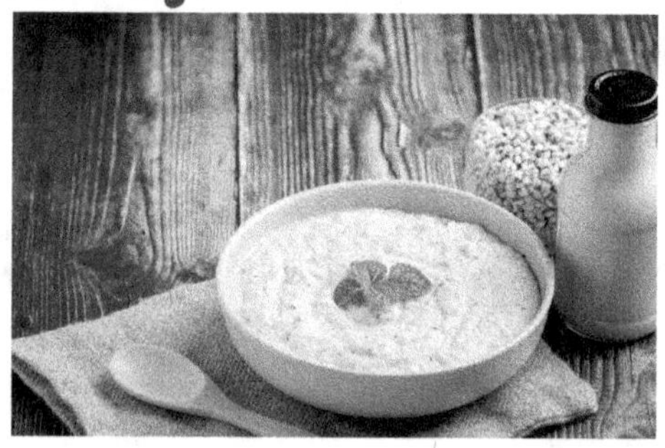

Millet porridge is a cozy dish made by cooking millet grains in water or milk until soft and creamy. It has a nutty taste and a smooth, thick texture like porridge. People often add cinnamon or cardamom for extra flavor and sweeten it with honey or sugar. It's full of nutrients, gentle on the stomach, and loved around the world for its nourishing goodness and comforting feel.

Preparation time

- Ready In:30 mins

Ingredients:

- ⅓ cup millet
- ¾ cup water
- ½ cup skim milk or 1/2 cup soy milk
- ¼ tsp ground cinnamon
- ½ tsp vanilla extract

Pinch of salt

- 2 tbsp raisins (adjust to taste)
- Honey or sweetener, to taste

Directions:

1. In a small saucepan, combine millet, water, milk, cinnamon, vanilla extract, salt, and raisins.

2. Bring to a boil over medium-high heat.

3. Reduce heat to low, cover, and simmer without stirring for 25 minutes.

4. If the liquid isn't fully absorbed after 25 minutes, cook for an additional 3-5 minutes, partially covered.

5. Remove from heat.

6. Sweeten with honey or your preferred sweetener.

7. Serve warm.

Nutrition Facts

- Serving Size: 1 portion (391 grams)
- Servings Per Recipe:1

Amount Per Serving

- Calories: 369
- % Daily Value
- Calories from Fat: 28 grams (8% DV)
- Total Fat: 3.2 grams (4% DV)

- Saturated Fat: 0.7 grams (3% DV)
- Cholesterol: 2.5 milligrams (0% DV)
- Sodium: 238.7 milligrams (9% DV)
- Total Carbohydrate: 71.8 grams (23% DV)
- Dietary Fiber: 6.7 grams (26% DV)
- Sugars: 12 grams
- Protein: 12.8 grams (2

6. Avocado Toast

Avocado toast is a popular dish made by spreading creamy avocado on toasted bread, usually sourdough or whole grain. It's seasoned with salt, pepper, and sometimes chili flakes. People often add toppings like cherry tomatoes, poached eggs, or microgreens to create a mix of flavors and textures—crunchy toast with creamy avocado. It's loved for being easy to make, good for you, and great for breakfast or a quick meal.

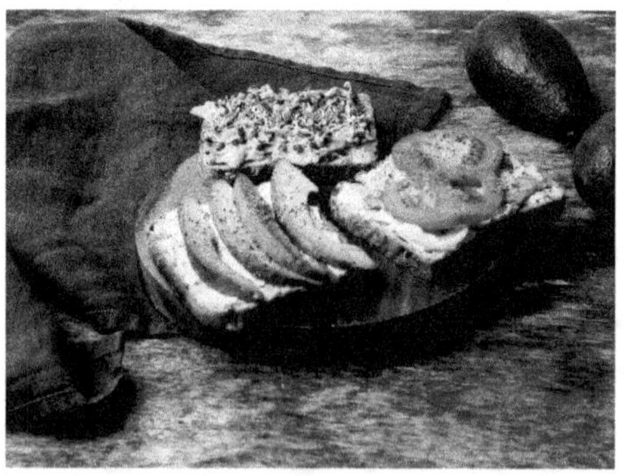

Here's how to create exceptional avocado toast

1) Pick ripe Hass avocados that feel slightly soft when squeezed. Cut away any bruised areas.

2) Use thick slices of whole grain bread and toast until golden for a crispy base.

3) Mash avocados separately until smooth in a bowl or on a plate to keep the toast intact.

4) Add a pinch of salt to each half of mashed avocado and sprinkle with flaky sea salt for extra taste.

Preparation time

- Preparation:
- 3 minutes
- Cooking:
- 2 minutes
- Total:
- 5 minutes
- Yield: 1 slice
- Category: Breakfast, Snack
- Method: Toasted

- 1 slice of thick whole-wheat bread
- 1/2 ripe avocado
- Pinch of salt
- Optional: Any toppings you like

Instructions

1. Toast a slice of bread until it's golden and crisp.

2. Remove the pit from the avocado. Scoop out the flesh into a bowl and mash it with a fork until smooth.

3. Add a small pinch of salt to the mashed avocado, adjusting to taste.

4. Spread the mashed avocado on the toasted bread. Enjoy it plain or add toppings like a sprinkle of sea salt.

5. To make it gluten-free, use gluten-free bread like Canyon Bakehouse 7-Grain Bread from Natural Grocers.

Nutrition Facts

- Serving Size: 1 slice of whole grain toast with half an avocado and a pinch of sea salt (no other toppings)
- Calories: 237
- Total Fat: 15.8g (20% DV)
- Saturated Fat: 2.4g
- Trans Fat: 0.3g
- Polyunsaturated Fat: 2g
- Monounsaturated Fat: 10.3g
- Cholesterol: 0mg
- Sodium: 413.3mg (18% DV)
- Total Carbohydrate: 21.4g (8% DV)
- Dietary Fiber: 8.6g (31% DV)
- Sugars: 2.1g
- Protein: 6.1g (12% DV)

<u>Vitamins and Minerals (% DV)</u>

- Vitamin A: 1%
- Vitamin C: 11%
- Calcium: 3%
- Iron: 7%
- Vitamin D: 0%
- Magnesium: 13%
- Potassium: 12%
- Zinc: 11%
- Phosphorus: 10%
- Thiamin (B1): 13%
- Riboflavin (B2): 16%
- Niacin (B3): 20%
- Vitamin B6: 19%
- Folic Acid (B9): 24%
- Vitamin B12: 20%
- Vitamin E: 15%
- Vitamin K: 29%

7. Coconut Yogurt Parfait

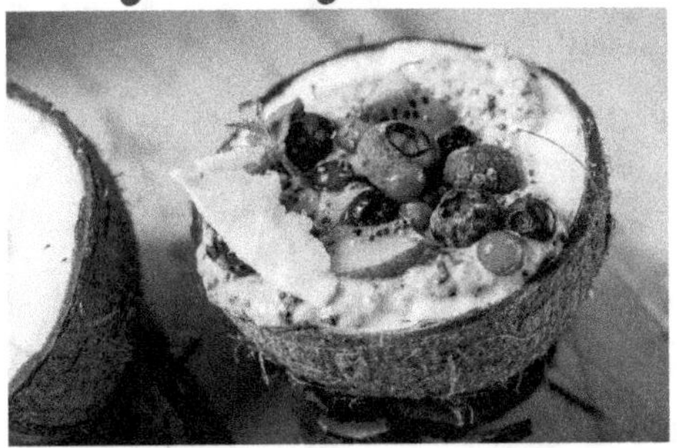

Enjoy our Coconut Yogurt Parfait, a mix of creamy coconut yogurt with tropical fruits, crunchy granola, and honey. Each bite is a blend of smooth coconut yogurt, sweet mangoes, tangy pineapple, and topped with toasted coconut flakes. It's a delicious treat that feels like a sunny island escape in every spoonful.

Parfait is a layered dish served in a glass or bowl. It originated in France and involves cooking cream, eggs, sugar, and syrup to make a smooth, custard-like mixture that's easier to prepare than ice cream. In the United States, parfaits are like sundaes with layers of ice cream or cream, fruits, nuts, syrups, and sometimes whipped cream. Yogurt is often used instead of cream or ice cream for a healthier option. Parfaits can be enjoyed as delicious treats or healthy snacks, depending on what ingredients are used.

Preparation Time:

- 5 minutes
- Total Time:
- 5 minutes
- Yield: Makes 2 parfaits

Ingredients:

- 2 cups (300 g) coconut yogurt
- 1 cup (30 ml) assorted fresh fruits
- 1 cup (5 ml) crunchy granola

Instructions:

1. Prepare each part separately. If making your own coconut yogurt or granola, start with those.

2. Layer the parfaits. Put half of the coconut yogurt into a clear glass first. Add half of the fresh fruits, then half of the granola. Repeat

with another layer of yogurt, fruits, and granola. Make sure each layer spreads to the edges of the glass for a nice look.

3. Serve right away.

4. To store, you can keep prepared coconut yogurt parfaits in the fridge for up to 5 days. For the crunchiest granola, store yogurt, fruits, and granola separately in sealed containers. Or, assemble the parfaits without granola and add it just before serving to keep it crispy.

Nutritional Information (Per Serving):

- Calories: About 530 kcal
- Total Fat: 46g
- Saturated Fat: 20g
- Total Carbohydrates: 71g
- Dietary Fiber: 13g
- Sugars: 38g
- Protein: 8g

8. Quinoa Porridge

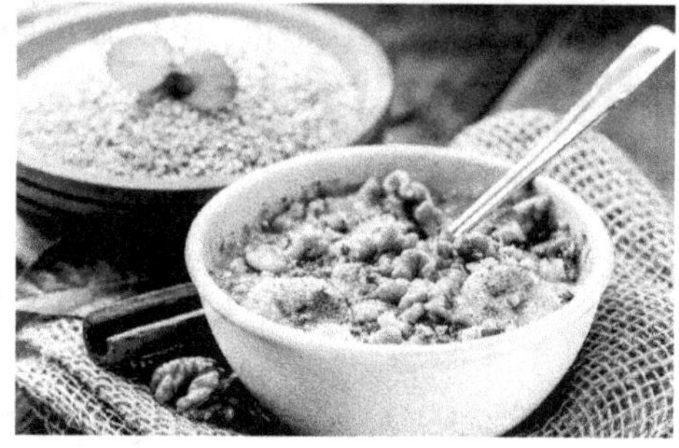

Quinoa Porridge is a healthy breakfast made by cooking quinoa in milk or water until it's soft and creamy. It has a slightly nutty taste with a hint of sweetness. You can top it with fresh fruits, nuts, honey, or cinnamon. It's packed with protein, fiber, and vitamins, making it a great way to start your day feeling satisfied and balanced.

<u>*Preparation time*</u>

- Preparation:
- 5 minutes
- Cooking:
- 30 minutes
- Total:
- 35 minutes
- Servings: 3

<u>*Ingredients*</u>

- 1/2 cup quinoa
- 1/4 tsp cinnamon powder
- 1 and 1/2 cups almond milk
- 1/2 cup water
- 2 tbsp brown sugar
- 1 tsp vanilla extract (optional)
- A pinch of salt

Direction:

First, heat a pan on medium heat. Put in the quinoa and cinnamon. Stir lots for about 3 minutes until it smells good. Add almond milk, water, and vanilla. Mix in brown sugar and a little salt. Let it boil, then turn down the heat and simmer gently for about 25 minutes until it's thick and the quinoa is soft. If it gets too thick, add more water. Stir sometimes, especially at the end, so it doesn't stick. To make it tastier, you can add fruits, nuts, or honey on top when you serve it.

Nutritional value

1. serving:
2. 173 Calories
3. 3 grams of Fat
4. 31 grams of Carbohydrates
5. 4 grams of Protein

9. Vegan Breakfast Cookies

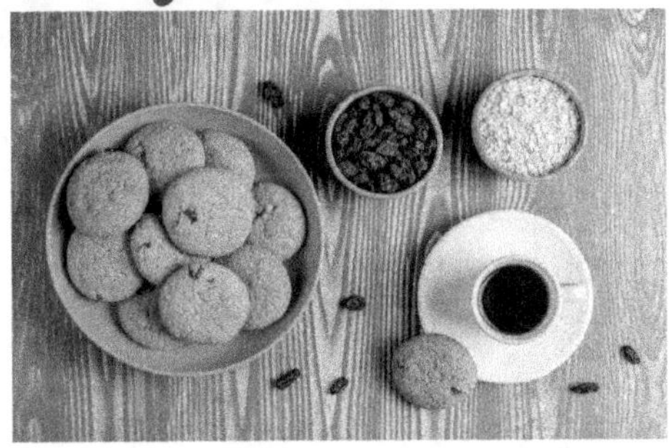

These vegan breakfast cookies are full of healthy ingredients like oats, nuts, seeds, and dried fruits. They're crunchy, sweet, and great for a nutritious breakfast. These cookies are tasty and easy to grab for a quick energy boost in the morning. Enjoy them with coffee or as a snack that satisfies your hunger and tastes great.

Preparation time

- Prep Time:
- 10 minutes
- Cook Time:
- 17 minutes
- Total Time:
- 27 minutes

- Servings: 26 cookies
- Course: Breakfast, Dessert, Snack
- Cuisine:Gluten-Free, Vegan
- Freezer Friendly: Up to 1 month
- Storage: 3-4 days

Ingredients:

- 2 tbsp flaxseed meal
- 5 tbsp water
- 2 medium ripe bananas
- 1/2 cup natural peanut butter (smooth or crunchy)
- 1/2 tsp baking powder
- 1/2 tsp baking soda
- 2 tbsp melted refined coconut oil (or avocado oil)
- 3 tbsp agave nectar or maple syrup (use honey if not vegan)
- Pinch of sea salt (adjust to taste)
- 1 tsp vanilla extract
- 1 1/2 cups gluten-free rolled oats
- 1/2 cup almond meal

- 1/2 cup oat flour (ground from gluten-free oats)
- 1/2 cup dairy-free semisweet or dark chocolate chips
- 3 tbsp raw walnuts, lightly crushed (or other nuts)

Instructions:

1. Preheat your oven to 350°F (176°C).

2. In a large bowl, mix flaxseed meal and water. Let it sit for 5 minutes until thickened.

3. Mash bananas into the flaxseed mixture until smooth.

4. Stir in peanut butter, baking powder, baking soda, melted coconut oil, agave nectar (or maple syrup), salt, and vanilla extract until well combined.

5. Add oats, almond meal, and oat flour. Mix until evenly incorporated.

6. Gently fold in chocolate chips and crushed walnuts.

7. Refrigerate dough for 5 minutes to firm up.

8. Drop spoonfuls of dough onto a lightly greased baking sheet.

9. Bake for 15-17 minutes until cookies are lightly golden brown.

10. Cool on the baking sheet for a few minutes, then transfer to a wire rack to cool completely.

11. Store cookies in an airtight container at room temperature for 3-4 days. For longer storage, refrigerate or freeze.

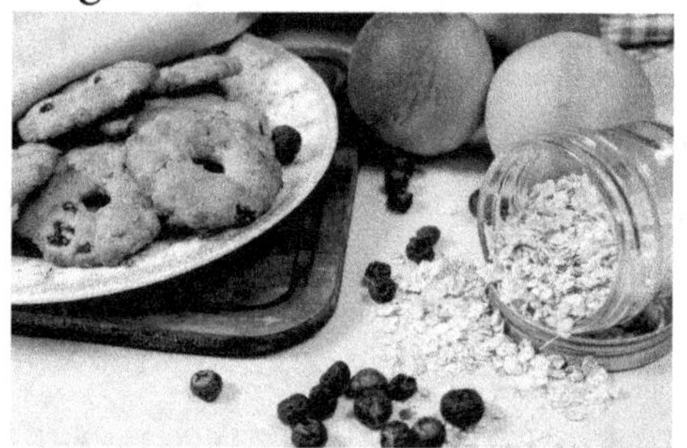

Notes:

- These cookies are high in fiber and protein, perfect for a satisfying snack.
- Customize with dried fruits, seeds, or your favorite nuts.
- Ensure ingredients are at room temperature for best results.

Enjoy these easy Nutty Banana Peanut Butter Cookies for a tasty treat any time!

10. Vegan Banana Pancakes

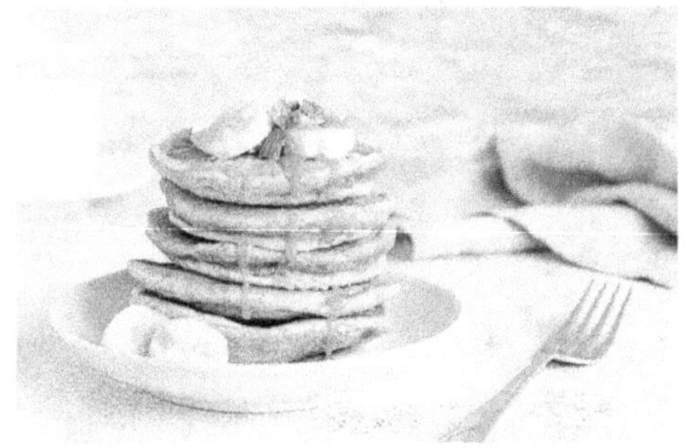

Vegan Banana Pancakes are a healthy, plant-based twist on regular pancakes. They're made with mashed ripe bananas for sweetness and a soft texture. You can use whole wheat or gluten-free flour for a wholesome base. They're flavored with vanilla and cinnamon, giving off a cozy smell when cooking. Top them with maple syrup, fresh berries, or sliced bananas for a tasty breakfast or brunch. These pancakes are a nourishing way to start your day, free from animal products and full of good ingredients.

Here are the nutrition facts per serving for this dairy-free, egg-free, vegan, and vegetarian option:

Preparation time
- Prep:10 mins
- Cook:12 mins

Nutritional Information
- Calories: 94 kcal
- Fat: 4g (low)
- Saturated Fat: 0g
- Carbohydrates: 14g
- Sugars: 6g (low)
- Fiber: 1g
- Protein: 1g
- Salt: 0.2g

<u>*Ingredients:*</u>

- 1 large ripe banana (about 150g)
- 2 tbsp golden caster sugar
- ¼ tsp fine salt
- 2 tbsp vegetable oil, plus more for cooking
- 120g self-raising flour
- ½ tsp baking powder
- 150ml oat, almond, or soya milk
- Syrup, sliced banana, and berries, to serve (optional)

Instructions

<u>Step 1: Make the Batter</u>

Mash the ripe banana in a bowl until smooth. Add sugar, salt, and vegetable oil. Mix well. Stir in the flour and baking powder until fully combined. Make a well in the center and slowly whisk in the milk until you get a thick batter.

Step 2: Cook the Pancakes

Heat a bit of oil in a frying pan over medium heat. Pour about 2 tablespoons of batter for each pancake into the pan. Cook for 2-3 minutes on each side until golden brown.

Step 3: Serve

Serve the pancakes warm with syrup. Add sliced bananas and berries for extra flavor and a nice presentation.

Tips:

- Let the batter rest a few minutes for fluffier pancakes.
- Try different toppings like nuts, whipped cream, or chocolate chips.
- Store leftovers in the fridge and reheat in a toaster or microwave.

Enjoy these delicious banana pancakes for breakfast or as a tasty snack!

11. Anti-Inflammatory Smoothie

"Boost your day with our Anti-Inflammatory Smoothie, made to soothe and refresh. It's packed with fresh turmeric, ginger, spinach, and antioxidant-rich berries to help reduce inflammation and support your body. Enjoy its delicious flavor anytime – perfect for starting your day or after a workout. Feel good with every sip, promoting a healthy and vibrant lifestyle effortlessly."

Ingredients:

- ¾ cup diced pear (with skin)
- 2 tsp freshly grated ginger
- ¾ cup fresh spinach
- ¾ cup oat milk (or any milk you like)
- 2 tsp hemp or chia seeds
- 1 tsp honey or maple syrup (optional)
- 1 cup ice cubes

1. Put pear, ginger, spinach, oat milk, and seeds in a blender.
2. Blend until smooth.
3. Add ½ cup ice and blend until creamy.
4. Taste and add honey or maple syrup for sweetness if desired.

Notes:

- Makes about 1.5 servings.
- You can use any milk you prefer instead of oat milk.
- Substitute arugula for spinach if you're sensitive to histamine.
- Any sweet pear variety works well, like Bartlett pears.

Nutrition:

- Serving Size: 1 smoothie
- Calories: 209 kcal
- Carbs: 27g

- Protein: 13g
- Fat: 6g
- Fiber: 4g
- Sugars: 13g
- Vitamins and Minerals: Includes Vitamin A, C, Calcium, Iron

Conclusion

"To sum up, we've looked at a great variety of breakfast recipes to make your mornings better. Whether you like traditional favorites or new ideas, these dishes will please everyone. They're perfect for quick, healthy bites or relaxed weekend brunches. Enjoy starting your day with good ingredients and delicious flavors. Next, in Chapter 4, we'll explore Lunch and Dinner Ideas to keep your day going strong."

Chapters 4 : Lunch and Dinner Ideas

Chapter 4 is all about delicious meals you can enjoy any time of day. It has quick and healthy lunch ideas and filling dinners that make everyone happy. You'll find easy recipes with different flavors to suit different tastes and diets. Whether you like colorful salads, cozy soups, or tasty main dishes, this chapter gives you simple instructions and tips to make cooking easier. It's all about making your meals special with these great lunch and dinner ideas!

4.1 "Tasty Lunch Ideas:

1.Flavorful Buddha Bowls

These colorful bowls are filled with fresh and healthy ingredients for a satisfying meal. They include grains like quinoa or brown rice, mixed with veggies such as roasted sweet potatoes, bell peppers, and greens. Buddha Bowls look great and taste delicious! You can add grilled chicken, tofu, or chickpeas on top, and finish with a tasty dressing or tahini sauce. They're perfect if you want a nutritious and tasty meal that keeps you feeling good!

Preparation Time:

- 15 minutes
- Cooking Time:
- 20 minutes
- Total Time:
- 35 minutes
- Serves: 4

Ingredients:

- 1 large yam, cut into small cubes
- Drizzle of avocado oil
- 1 purple daikon or 2 red radishes, thinly sliced
- 2 medium parsnips, peeled and chopped
- 1 cup thinly sliced purple cabbage
- Juice of one lime

- 8 chard leaves, finely chopped
- 2 cups cooked wild rice or millet
- 1 cup cooked black beans or chickpeas
- ¾ cup kimchi or fermented pickles
- 2 tablespoons flax seeds or chia seeds
- Golden Almond Sauce, for serving
- Sprouts or edible flowers, optional
- Himalayan salt and cracked black pepper

Additional Tips:

1. Prepare Ahead: Roast the yams ahead of time and store them in the fridge for quicker meal prep.

2. Texture Variation: Try cutting the daikon into noodle-like spirals for a fun twist.

3. Colorful Crunch: Add shredded beets or orange bell peppers for more color and crunchiness.

4.*Boost Protein:* Include grilled tofu or tempeh cubes to increase the protein content.

5.*Garnish Ideas:* Sprinkle toasted almonds or pumpkin seeds on top for a crunchy finish.

Enjoy making this colorful and nutritious bowl!

Instructions

1. Preheat your oven to 400°F and line a baking sheet with parchment paper.

2. Coat sweet potatoes with olive oil, salt, and pepper. Spread them on the baking sheet and bake for 20 minutes until crispy and golden.

3. Slice radishes thinly using a mandoline if available. Use a peeler to make carrot ribbons. Mix these with shredded cabbage and a squeeze of lemon juice. Set aside.

4. In a bowl, toss kale with lemon juice and a pinch of salt. Massage until it softens and halves in volume.

5. Build bowls with brown rice, chickpeas, kale, carrots, radishes, cabbage, roasted sweet potatoes, sauerkraut, sesame seeds, and optional microgreens. Season with salt and pepper, and serve with Turmeric Tahini Sauce.

Ingredients:

- Quinoa (1 cup, cooked)
- Mixed greens (1 cup)
- Roasted sweet potatoes (1 medium)
- Chickpeas (1/2 cup, cooked)
- Avocado (1/2 medium)
- Cherry tomatoes (1/2 cup)
- Cucumber slices (1/2 cup)
- Hummus (2 tbsp)
- Olive oil (1 tbsp, for dressing)

<u>*Nutritional Value:*</u>

- Calories: About 550-600 kcal
- Protein: 15-20 grams
- Carbohydrates: About 70-80 grams
- Fiber: 15-20 grams
- Fat: About 20-25 grams

- Vitamins and Minerals: Provides good amounts of Vitamin A, Vitamin C, Vitamin K, folate, potassium, magnesium, and iron.

2. Hearty Vegan Soups

"Hearty vegan soups are comforting bowls full of healthy ingredients like vegetables, beans, and grains. They're flavorful, seasoned with herbs and spices, and packed with nutrients like protein from beans, fiber from veggies, and important vitamins and minerals. Perfect for cold days, they're warm and delicious, making them a great choice for adding plant-based nutrition to your diet."

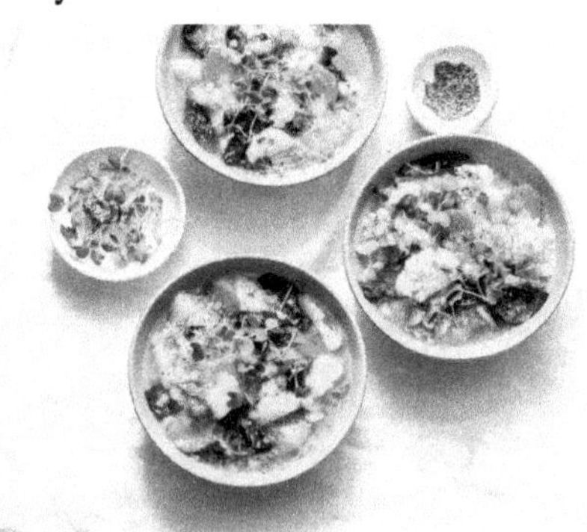

This recipe is for 4 to 6 servings. It takes 20 minutes to prepare and 90 minutes to cook.

Ingredients:

- 2 tbsp / 30 ml extra virgin olive oil (or vegetable stock for a no-oil option)
- 1 large onion, finely chopped
- 6 garlic cloves, finely chopped
- 2 sprigs fresh rosemary, finely chopped or 1 tsp dried rosemary
- 4 sprigs fresh thyme, leaves picked or ½ tsp dried thyme
- 2 celery stalks, roughly chopped
- 2 carrots, roughly chopped
- 1½ tsp sweet smoked paprika
- 1¼ tsp salt, adjust to taste
- ½ tsp black pepper
- ¼ tsp red pepper flakes (optional), adjust to taste
- 2 x 400 g / 14 oz cans whole peeled tomatoes*
- 2 bay leaves (preferably fresh)

- 500 g / 17½ oz (about 5 medium) potatoes, scrubbed and cubed (about ¾" dice)
- 250 g / 8¾ oz (½ small) savoy cabbage, finely shredded

Instructions

1. Heat olive oil in a large pot over medium heat. If using the no-oil option, start with vegetable stock and add chopped onion.

2. Add chopped onion to the pot and cook until soft, about 5 minutes.

3. Stir in garlic, rosemary, and thyme, and cook for another 2-3 minutes until fragrant.

4. Add chopped celery and carrots, and cook for 5-10 minutes, stirring often.

5. Stir in smoked paprika, salt, black pepper, and red pepper flakes (if using).

6. Add canned tomatoes to the pot, crushing them with a spoon or masher.

7. Pour in 500 ml / 2 cups of water and add bay leaves. Cover and simmer for about 45 minutes, stirring occasionally. Add more water if needed.

8. Once tomatoes break down and soup thickens, add another 250 ml / 1 cup of water if needed, and simmer for 15 minutes.

9. Pour in another 750 ml / 3 cups of water and add potatoes. Simmer for 10 minutes.

10. Add shredded cabbage and simmer for another 5 minutes until potatoes are tender and cabbage is cooked.

11. Taste and adjust seasoning. Add sugar if tomatoes are too tangy.

12. For best flavor, let the soup sit overnight before serving. Adjust consistency with water when reheating.

13. Serve hot, optionally garnished with vegan pesto.

Nutritional value

- Calories: 255 (13% of daily recommended intake)
- Sugars: 13 grams (15% of daily recommended intake)
- Fats: 8 grams (11% of daily recommended intake)
- Saturated fats: 1 gram (6% of daily recommended intake)

- Proteins: 7 grams (14% of daily recommended intake)
- Carbohydrates: 42 grams (16% of daily recommended intake)
- Amounts are per serving

3. Vegan Sushi Rolls

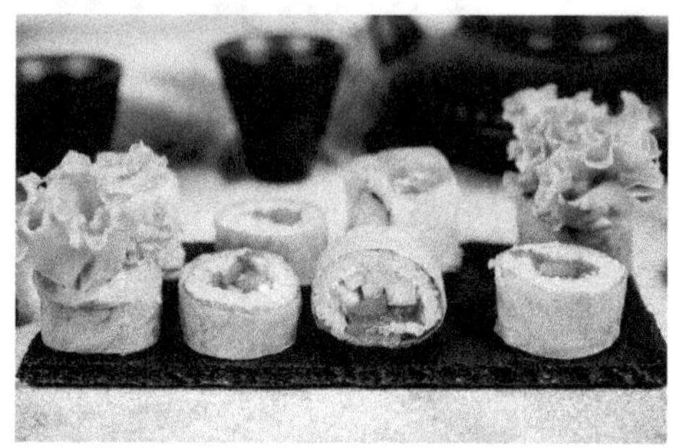

Vegan sushi rolls are packed with delicious flavors and textures, made without any animal products. They include sushi rice wrapped in seaweed, filled with fresh cucumber, creamy avocado, tangy pickled radish, and soft tofu. Topped with sesame seeds and served with soy sauce or wasabi, they're full of tasty umami. These rolls are perfect for plant-based diets and show how sushi can be both artistic and cruelty-free.

You can Make vegan sushi with Chioggia beets as a tuna substitute. Roast the beets until tender, then soak them in a mix of tamari, rice vinegar, sesame oil, and ginger. Spread sushi rice on nori sheets, add beets, cucumber, and avocado, and roll tightly with a bamboo mat. Slice and enjoy with sesame seeds, pickled ginger, and sriracha mayo if desired!

Preparation Time:

- 30 minutes
- Cooking Time:
- 1 hour
- Serves: 4

Ingredients:

- For the beet marinade:
- 2 pink Chioggia beets, thinly sliced
- Olive oil, for drizzling
- 1 tbsp rice vinegar
- 1 tbsp soy sauce
- ½ tbsp sesame oil
- ½ tsp grated ginger
- Pinch of sea salt

For the seasoned rice:

- 1 cup short-grain white rice
- 2 tbsp rice vinegar
- 1 tbsp sugar
- 1 tsp sea salt

For assembling the rolls:

- 4 nori sheets
- 1 Persian cucumber, thinly sliced
- 1 avocado, thinly sliced
- Sesame seeds, for sprinkling
- Soy sauce, for serving
- Pickled ginger, for serving
- Optional: Vegan mayo and sriracha

Instructions

1. Preheat your oven to 400°F. Wrap whole beets individually in foil after drizzling each with olive oil and sprinkling salt. Roast them on a baking sheet for 45 to 60 minutes until they're soft and can be easily pierced with a fork. Let

them cool, peel off the skins under running water, and slice into thin strips.

2. In a small bowl, mix rice vinegar, tamari, sesame oil, and ginger. Add the beet slices, toss well, and let them marinate for 15 minutes.

3. Cook rice as per package instructions, then mix it with vinegar, sugar, and salt.

4. To assemble rolls, place a nori sheet on a bamboo mat with the shiny side down. Spread rice on the lower two-thirds of the nori, then add rows of beet, cucumber, and avocado slices near the bottom edge. Roll tightly using the bamboo mat, press gently to shape, and repeat for remaining sheets.

5. Use a sharp knife to cut the rolls into pieces, wiping the knife between cuts. Sprinkle sesame seeds on top and serve with tamari, pickled ginger, and a mix of vegan mayo and sriracha on the side, if desired.

<u>**Nutritional value**</u>

- Calories: 300 kcal
- Fat: 7g
- Saturated Fat: 1g
- Unsaturated Fat: 6g
- Sodium: 600mg
- Carbohydrates: 54g
- Fiber: 6g
- Sugars: 3g
- Protein: 8g

Note that actual values may vary depending on the ingredients used.

4. Peach Burrata Salad

Peach Burrata Salad has ripe peaches, creamy burrata cheese, and fresh greens like arugula. It's dressed with tangy vinaigrette for a tasty mix of sweet and savory. This salad is fresh and satisfying, perfect for a light meal on a sunny day.

Gluten-free, low-sodium, vegan dish.

<u>Preparation time:</u>
- 20 minutes
- Serves: 4
- Total calories: 264 kcal

<u>Ingredients:</u>
- A generous handful of peppery arugula
- 6 ripe strawberries, thinly sliced
- 1-2 small, juicy mangoes, thinly sliced
- 1 ball of creamy mozzarella, torn into rustic pieces

Basil Bliss Dressing:

- 2 cups fresh basil leaves
- 1 small shallot, peeled
- 1 small garlic clove
- ½ cup extra virgin olive oil
- 2 tablespoons clear apple cider vinegar
- ½ teaspoon sea salt
- ½ teaspoon freshly ground mixed peppercorns

Instructions:

1. Finely chop shallot and garlic in a food processor.

2. Add basil leaves, olive oil, vinegar, salt, and pepper. Blend until smooth.

3. In a large bowl, layer arugula, strawberries, mangoes, and torn mozzarella.

4. Drizzle basil bliss dressing generously over the salad and sprinkle with extra ground peppercorns.

Tips:

- Toss ingredients with dressing just before serving for best flavor.
- Store dressing in the fridge for up to a week.
- Substitute spinach or mixed greens for arugula for variety.

Nutrition Facts:

- Serving Size: 1 plate
- Calories: 264 kcal
- Carbohydrates: 5g
- Protein: 1g
- Fat: 27g
- Saturated Fat: 4g
- Cholesterol: 1mg
- Sodium: 292mg
- Potassium: 135mg
- Fiber: 1g
- Sugars: 4g
- Vitamin A: 762IU
- Vitamin C: 15mg
- Calcium: 29mg

- Iron: 1mg

Enjoy this vibrant summertime salad packed with flavors and wholesome ingredients!

5. Boursin Stuffed Mushrooms

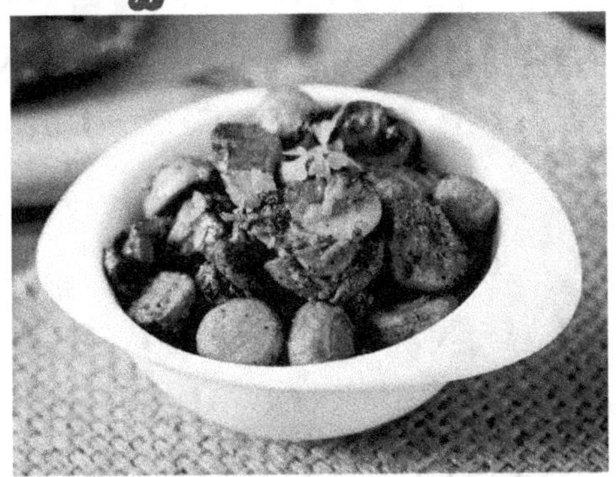

Boursin Stuffed Mushrooms combine earthy mushroom flavors with creamy Boursin cheese. They have a savory, creamy taste with herbs and spices. These mushrooms are carefully stuffed and baked until golden brown, making them delicious to eat. Whether you serve them at a fancy dinner or as a comfy snack, they're sure to be enjoyed for their tasty mix of flavors and textures.

Ingredients

1. Choose your favorite vegan Boursin-style cheese flavor, like Garlic and Herbs, Shallot and Chive, Black Pepper, or Basil. Look for

dairy-free options at health food stores or vegan sections of supermarkets. You can also use vegan cream cheese or other plant-based cheeses you have.

2. Pick any type of mushrooms, but white button mushrooms or baby bellas are recommended for their taste and texture. Larger white mushrooms work especially well. Find affordable ones at places like Costco or local farmers' markets.

3. Spread the vegan Boursin-style cheese generously over the mushrooms.

4. Optional: Add chopped fresh Italian parsley and freshly ground pepper for extra flavor.

Enjoy your easy vegan dish!

How to Clean Mushrooms

For great cheese stuffed mushrooms, avoid soaking them in water. It can make them soggy and affect how they roast. Instead, use a slightly damp paper towel to gently wipe off any dirt. This keeps them dry and perfect for cooking!

Preparation Time:

- 5 minutes
- Cooking Time:
- 15 minutes
- Total Time:
- 20 minutes
- Servings: 6
- Calories: 110 kcal

Ingredients:

- 24 oz large white mushrooms
- 5.2 oz package of Boursin Garlic and Herb cheese
- 2 tablespoons chopped fresh parsley (optional)

- Salt and pepper to taste

Instructions:

1. Preheat your oven to 425°F. Clean the mushrooms by wiping them with a damp paper towel. Remove the stems and set the caps on a parchment-lined baking sheet.

2. Fill each mushroom cap with 2-3 teaspoons of Boursin cheese. Place them back on the baking sheet and bake at 425°F. Smaller mushrooms bake for 12-13 minutes, larger ones for 15-16 minutes, until the cheese is lightly browned and mushrooms are tender.

3. Transfer the baked mushroom caps to a serving plate. Sprinkle with parsley and cracked black pepper. Taste and add salt if desired.

Notes:

- Typically serves 3-4 mushrooms per person, depending on size.

- Best results with Boursin flavors like Garlic and Herb, Black Pepper, Basil, or Shallot and Chive.
- Can be prepared ahead: stuff mushrooms, refrigerate, and bake when ready.
- Gluten-free; use dairy-free Boursin for a dairy-free option (not suitable for all elimination diets).
- For lower sodium, use herbed goat cheese or cream cheese instead of Boursin.

Nutrition (per serving of 4 mushrooms):

- Calories: 110
- Carbohydrates: 6g
- Protein: 5g
- Fat: 9g (Saturated Fat: 5g)
- Cholesterol: 27mg
- Sodium: 139 mg
- Potassium: 361mg
- Fiber: 1g
- Sugar: 2g
- Vitamin C: 2mg

- Calcium: 3mg
- Iron: 1mg

6. Butter Lettuce Salad

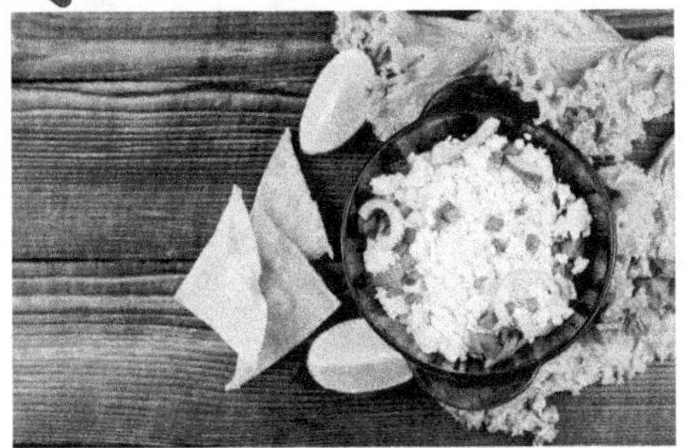

Butter lettuce is famous for its smooth and velvety texture, which is why it's called "butter." It's also known as butterhead or Boston bibb lettuce and is loved for its soft leaves and mild taste. Mixing it with crispy things like thinly sliced radishes not only gives a nice texture difference but also makes the dish taste even better.

This recipe is free from gluten and dairy, and it's good for the brain.

<u>Preparation Time:</u>

- 15 minutes
- Total Time:
- 15 minutes
- Servings: 4
- Calories: 144 kcal

<u>Ingredients:</u>

1. Fresh butter lettuce salad:

- 2-3 heads of butter lettuce (or bibb lettuce)
- A bunch of fresh chives
- 5-6 radishes, thinly sliced
- Freshly ground black pepper and sea salt to taste

2. Dijon dressing:

- 3 tbsp distilled white vinegar
- 4 tsp Dijon mustard
- 1 tbsp honey
- 1 tbsp finely chopped shallot
- 1/4 cup extra virgin olive oil

Instructions:

1. Separate the butter lettuce leaves, wash, and pat them dry.
2. Mix vinegar, Dijon mustard, honey, and shallot in a bowl. Gradually whisk in olive oil until smooth.
3. Toss lettuce with 2-3 tbsp of dressing, adjusting to taste. Arrange on a platter.
4. Top with chives, radishes, salt, and pepper.

Notes:

- Butter lettuce is also known as Boston or bibb lettuce.
- Optional additions include goat cheese, toasted sunflower seeds, or pepitas.
- Fresh chives are best; avoid substitutes.
- Use white wine vinegar if distilled white vinegar is unavailable.

<u>*Nutritional Information (per serving):*</u>

- Calories: 144 kcal
- Carbs: 5 g
- Protein: 1 g
- Fat: 14 g
- Sat. Fat: 2 g
- Polyunsat. Fat: 2 g
- Monounsat. Fat: 10 g
- Sodium: 58 mg
- Potassium: 219 mg
- Fiber: 1 g
- Sugar: 4 g
- Vitamin A: 2741 IU
- Vitamin C: 4 mg
- Calcium: 35 mg
- Iron: 1 mg

7.Sweet Potato Stew

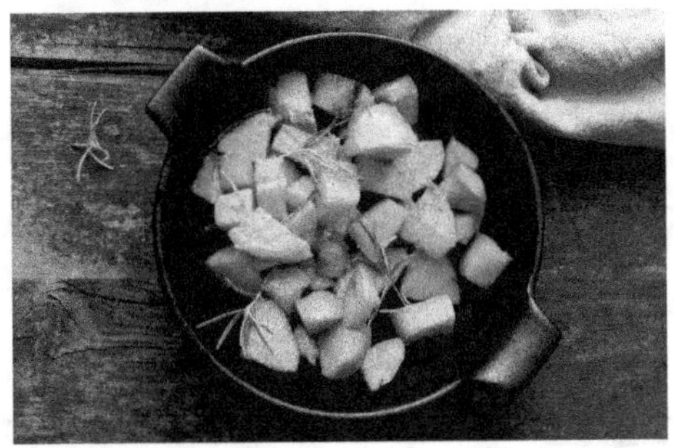

Sweet Potato Stew is a warm and comforting dish made with soft sweet potatoes, mixed with tasty veggies like carrots, onions, and celery. It's cooked in a flavorful broth with spices like cumin, paprika, and a touch of cinnamon. The sweet potatoes add a natural sweetness that goes well with the savory flavors, making it a satisfying meal. Top it with fresh parsley or cilantro for extra freshness. Sweet Potato Stew is nutritious and delicious, great for cozy dinners or sharing with family and friends.

Ingredient:

- **_Sweet potatoes:_** Approximately 1-2 large sweet potatoes, peeled and chopped (about 3 cups).

- **_Shallot:_** Provides a mild flavor akin to onions.

- **_Tomato paste:_** Adds thickness to the stew (optional, omit if sensitive).

- **_Spices:_** Curry powder, cumin, and ginger powder (ensure it's a curry blend, not Thai).

- **_Vegetable broth:_** Choose according to dietary preferences (onion-free options are available).

- **_Kale:_** Substitute with spinach if preferred.

- ***Sunflower seed butter:*** Adds creaminess (choose a sugar-free variety).

- ***Optional additions:*** Toasted sunflower seeds and cilantro for garnish.

Equipment

- A slow cooker or crockpot

Diet Type:

- Low-calorie
- low-lactose
- low-salt, vegan, vegetarian

Preparation Time:

- 10 minutes
- Cooking Time:
- 4 hours
- Total Time:
- 4 hours and 10 minutes
- Servings: 6

- Calories per Serving: 173

Ingredients:

- 3 cups sweet potatoes, peeled and diced
- 1 shallot, peeled and chopped
- 5 oz tomato paste
- 2 tsp curry powder
- 1 tsp ground cumin
- ½ tsp ground ginger
- 2 cups vegetable broth
- 1 tsp kosher salt
- 2 cups water
- 1 cup chopped kale
- ⅓ cup sunflower seed butter

Instructions:

For freezing:

1. Put sweet potatoes, shallot, tomato paste, curry powder, ginger, broth, and salt in a freezer bag. Freeze until ready.

<u>Cooking:</u>

1. In the slow cooker, combine all ingredients (except kale, water, and sunflower seed butter). Cook on high for 4 hours or low for 8 hours.

2. Thirty minutes before serving, add kale and water. Adjust seasoning. Just before serving, stir in sunflower seed butter.

3. For stovetop: Simmer ingredients (except kale and sunflower seed butter) in a covered pot for 30 mins. Add kale, then stir in sunflower seed butter before serving.

Tips:

- Add sunflower seed butter last to avoid separation.
- Garnish with cilantro and roasted sunflower seeds if desired.
- Use fresh ginger instead of ground.
- Choose low-sodium broth and unsalted sunflower seed butter.

<u>*Nutrition (per serving):*</u>

- Calories: 173
- Carbs: 24g
- Protein: 6g
- Fat: 7g
- Fiber: 4g
- Sugar: 6g
- Vitamins: A, C
- Minerals: Calcium, Iron

8. Mozzarella Alfredo Pasta Sauce

Explore a delicious variation of traditional pasta sauces with Mozzarella Alfredo Pasta Sauce. This creamy sauce swaps parmesan for mozzarella cheese, mixed with garlic, butter, and creamy goodness. It's perfect for turning plain fettuccine into a luxurious meal, ready in just 20 minutes. Great for relaxed dinners, it adds a smooth texture and rich flavor that makes any pasta dish taste gourmet.

Dietary Preference: Gluten-free, Low-sodium

Preparation Time:
- 5 minutes
- Cooking Time:
- 20 minutes
- Total Time:
- 25 minutes
- Servings: 4
- Calories per Serving: 539

Ingredients:

- 8 oz fettuccine pasta
- 3 tbsp butter
- 1 1/4 cups heavy cream
- 3 large cloves garlic
- 1 cup freshly shredded mozzarella (full-fat, low moisture)
- 1/8 tsp ground black pepper
- Kosher salt
- Optional: Italian parsley, nutmeg

Instructions:

1. Boil salted water in a large pot. Cook fettuccine according to package, then drain, saving 1 cup pasta water.

2. In a large pan, melt butter over medium heat. Add minced garlic, sauté for 1 minute. Pour in heavy cream, simmer until sauce thickens (5-6 mins).

3. Add cooked pasta to pan, toss to coat with sauce using tongs.

4. Stir in shredded mozzarella until melted. Add pasta water if needed for consistency.

5. Season with salt, pepper, and nutmeg. Garnish with parsley if desired.

6. Serve hot immediately. Cheese will thicken as it cools.

<u>Notes:</u>

- Use freshly grated, full-fat, low moisture mozzarella for best results. Brands like Boar's Head or Calabro are recommended.
- Tossing with tongs helps distribute sauce evenly.
- Use unsalted water for lower sodium. For gluten-free, use gluten-free pasta or serve over vegetables or chicken.

<u>*Nutrition (per serving):*</u>

- Calories: 539 kcal
- Carbs: 39g
- Protein: 20g
- Fat: 37g
- Sat Fat: 17g
- Cholesterol: 173mg
- Sodium: 279 mg
- Fiber: 2g
- Vit A: 1562 IU
- Vit C: 0.4mg
- Calcium: 268mg
- Iron: 1mg

9. Butternut Squash Soup

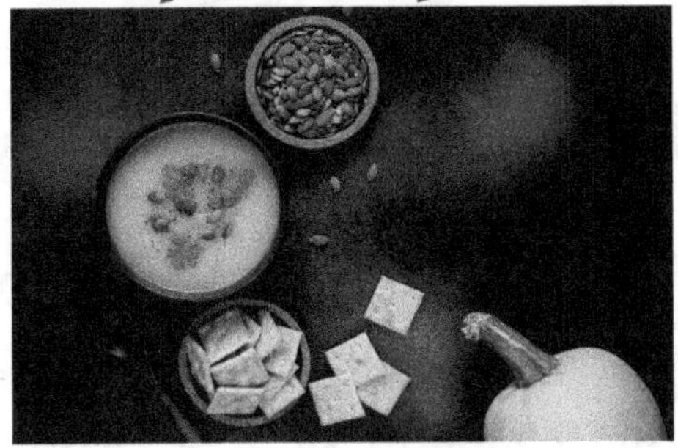

Enjoy the cozy comfort of homemade butternut squash soup made in an Instant Pot. This creamy soup blends the sweet flavor of roasted squash with aromatic spices for a smooth and nourishing treat, perfect for chilly autumn nights.

This Instant Pot butternut squash soup recipe is like Panera's Autumn Squash soup but vegan. It uses cubed squash, gentle shallots, and nutritious carrots. Sweetness comes from apple juice or cider, with vegetable broth for flavor. Maple syrup or honey adds more sweetness, while curry powder and ginger give it warmth. Top with pepitas for crunch. You can skip the cream for a lighter, vegan-friendly dish that's just as tasty.

Summary: This vegan twist on butternut squash soup skips dairy and uses vegan-friendly ingredients like vegetable broth. It's packed with autumn flavors and topped with crunchy pepitas.

Equipment:

- Choose either an Instant Pot, Slow Cooker, or Large Pot

This recipe is vegan and has low calories, fat, and salt. It takes 15 minutes to prepare and 10 minutes to cook, totaling 25 minutes. It serves 4 people and each serving has around 271 calories.

Ingredients:

- 2 tbsp olive oil
- 2 large shallots, roughly chopped
- 2 large carrots, roughly chopped

- 1 ½ lbs butternut squash, peeled, seeded, and cubed
- 3 cups vegetable broth
- 1 cup apple juice
- 1 tbsp honey or maple syrup
- 1 tbsp curry powder
- 2 tsp fresh minced ginger
- Salt and pepper, to taste
- ¼ cup heavy cream (optional)
- Toasted pepitas (pumpkin seeds), for topping

Instructions:

Instant Pot Method:

1. Heat olive oil in the Instant Pot using "saute" mode. Add shallots and carrots, cook until softened (1-2 minutes).

2. Add butternut squash, broth, apple juice, honey or maple syrup, curry powder, ginger, salt, and pepper.

3. Close the lid, seal the vent, and pressure cook for 10 minutes.

4. Allow natural release for 10-15 minutes. Carefully open the vent to release steam.

5. Blend the soup until smooth. Stir in cream if using, adjust seasoning.

6. Serve warm, topped with toasted pepitas.

Slow Cooker Method:

1. Combine all ingredients except cream in a slow cooker. Cook on low for 7-8 hours.

2. Blend soup until smooth. Stir in cream if desired, adjust seasoning.

3. Serve hot, garnished with toasted pepitas.

Stovetop Method:

1. Heat olive oil in a large pot over medium heat. Add shallots and carrots, sauté until softened (1-2 minutes).

2. Add butternut squash, broth, apple juice, honey, curry powder, ginger, salt, and pepper. Bring to a boil.

3. Reduce heat, cover, and simmer for 35-45 minutes until vegetables are tender.

4. Blend soup until smooth. Adjust seasoning and serve hot.

Recipe Notes:

- For a dairy-free option, skip the cream or use a substitute.
- Adjust curry powder to taste.
- Use low-sodium broth to reduce salt.
- Soup freezes well for up to 6 months.

Nutrition Information (per serving):

- Calories: 271 kcal
- Carbs: 40 g
- Protein: 4 g
- Fat: 13 g
- Sat Fat: 4 g
- Cholesterol: 17 mg
- Sodium: 37 mg
- Potassium: 842 mg
- Fiber: 6 g
- Sugar: 17 g
- Vitamins: A (23411 IU), C (39 mg)
- Calcium: 119 mg

- Iron: 2 mg

10. Fingerling Potato Salad

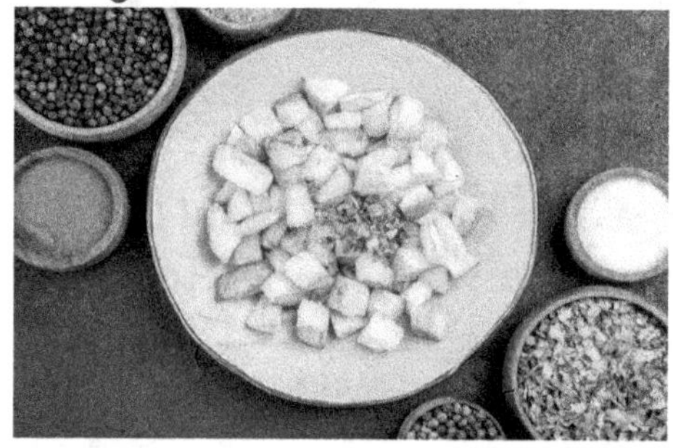

Our Fingerling Potato Salad mixes tender fingerling potatoes with a creamy, tangy sauce. We add fresh herbs, crunchy celery, and a touch of Dijon mustard for a perfect balance of flavors and textures. Enjoy it as a side dish or a light meal—it's a tasty blend of simple ingredients that's sure to satisfy.

Diet: Gluten-free, low salt, vegan, vegetarian

- 15 minutes
- Cook Time:
- 15 minutes
- Chilling Time:
- 1 hour
- Total Time:
- 1 hour 30 minutes
- Servings: 4
- Calories: 315 kcal

Ingredients:

- 2 pounds fingerling or small potatoes
- ⅓ cup mayonnaise
- 1 tablespoon Dijon mustard
- 1 tablespoon white vinegar
- 2 teaspoons apple juice
- 2 small stalks celery, diced
- 1 small shallot, finely chopped
- 1 teaspoon dried dill (or 1 tablespoon fresh)
- Salt and pepper to taste

Instructions:

1. Boil potatoes in salted water until fork-tender (about 10 minutes). Drain and let cool.

2. In a bowl, mix mayonnaise, Dijon mustard, vinegar, apple juice, celery, shallot, and dill.

3. Cut cooled potatoes into halves, add to the bowl, and gently mix until coated with dressing.

4. Season with salt and pepper to taste.

5. Chill for at least an hour before serving to enhance flavors.

Nutritional fact

- Calories: 315 kcal
- Carbohydrates: 42 g
- Protein: 5 g
- Fat: 14 g
- Saturated Fat: 2 g
- Cholesterol: 8 mg

- Sodium: 193 mg
- Potassium: 1028 mg
- Fiber: 6 g
- Sugar: 3 g
- Vitamin A: 189 IU
- Vitamin C: 47 mg
- Calcium: 40 mg
- Iron: 2 mg

Enjoy your simple and tasty Fingerling Potato Salad!

1. Caesar Salad Dressing without Anchovies

Absolutely! A Caesar salad dressing without anchovies keeps the classic flavors intact but with a twist. It mixes creamy mayonnaise, tangy Dijon mustard, fresh garlic, lemon juice for a zesty kick, and a bit of Worcestershire sauce for depth. This tasty dressing is great on crisp romaine lettuce, topped with Parmesan cheese and crunchy croutons, making a delicious and refreshing salad.

Equipment Needed:

- Whisk or immersion blender

- "Dietary: Suitable for diabetics, gluten-free, low-calorie, low-lactose, and low-salt.

Preparation Time:

- 10 minutes
- Total Time:
- 10 minutes
- Servings: 6 people
- Calories per serving: 144"

Ingredients:

- 2 tablespoons mayonnaise (use vegan mayo for a vegan option)
- 4-5 medium Kalamata or black olives, pitted and finely chopped
- 1 large garlic clove, minced
- 1 tablespoon distilled white vinegar or juice of ½ lemon
- 2 teaspoons Dijon mustard
- ⅓ cup extra virgin olive oil
- Freshly ground black pepper

For the Salad:

- 2-3 heads of romaine lettuce, washed and chopped
- Optional: homemade croutons

- Optional: Grilled or Baked Chicken or Shrimp

Instructions:

1. In a bowl, mix together mayonnaise, chopped olives, minced garlic, vinegar or lemon juice, and Dijon mustard until well combined.

2. Gradually pour in olive oil while whisking vigorously to create a smooth and creamy dressing. Add freshly ground black pepper to taste.

3. Alternatively, combine all ingredients in a jar and blend with an immersion blender until smooth. Be cautious not to over-blend to prevent separation of olive oil.

4. For grilled chicken, marinate for 2-3 hours. Grill over medium heat (about 425°F) for approximately 6 minutes per side or until the internal temperature reaches 165°F. Let the

chicken rest for 1-2 minutes before thinly slicing.

5. Toss chopped romaine lettuce with the dressing. Add croutons and grilled chicken or shrimp if desired. Adjust seasoning with salt to taste.

Notes:

- Kalamata, black, or Castelvetrano olives work well; capers are an alternative.
- Adjust ingredients for migraine-friendly diets by using distilled vinegar and olives packed in water.
- For re-introduction diets, use ½ lemon juice and optionally add ¼ cup freshly grated Parmesan.
- This dressing doubles as a great marinade for chicken or shrimp when grilling.

<u>**Nutrition (per serving):**</u>

- Calories: 144 kcal
- Carbohydrates: 0.4g
- Protein: 0.2g
- Fat: 16g
- Saturated Fat: 2g
- Polyunsaturated Fat: 3g
- Monounsaturated Fat: 10g
- Trans Fat: 0.01g
- Cholesterol: 2mg
- Sodium: 90mg
- Potassium: 7mg
- Fiber: 0.2g
- Sugar: 0.1g
- Vitamin A: 15IU
- Vitamin C: 0.2mg
- Calcium: 4mg
- Iron: 0.1mg

2. Vegan Pad Thai

Vegan Pad Thai is a delicious noodle dish with a mix of textures and flavors. It includes stir-fried rice noodles with crunchy vegetables like bean sprouts, bell peppers, and carrots. The noodles are flavored with a tangy sauce made from tamarind paste, soy sauce, and lime juice. Crushed peanuts add a nice crunch, while fresh cilantro and lime wedges give it a bright finish. Overall, Vegan Pad Thai offers a tasty balance of sweet, savory, and tangy tastes in every bite.

Preparation time:

- 10 minutes
- Cook time:
- 20 minutes
- Total time:
- 30 minutes
- Servings: 4

Ingredients:

- 7 ounces stir fry rice noodles
- 2-3 tablespoons vegetable oil
- 14.5 ounce block extra-firm tofu, cubed

Sauce:

- 4 tablespoons low sodium soy sauce
- 2 tablespoons rice vinegar
- 4 tablespoons pure maple syrup
- 2 tablespoons fresh lime juice
- 1 teaspoon Sriracha hot sauce

Vegetables:

- 1 cup julienne sliced carrots (about 3 carrots)
- 3 green onions, chopped

For serving:

- 2 limes, cut into wedges
- 1/2 cup chopped cilantro
- 1/2 cup crushed or chopped peanuts
- 1 cup mung bean sprouts (optional)

1. Cook the noodles: Boil them for 1 minute, then let soak for 5 minutes. Drain and rinse with cold water.

2. Make the sauce: Mix soy sauce, rice vinegar, maple syrup, lime juice, and Sriracha in a bowl.

3. Fry the tofu: Heat oil in a large pan over medium-high heat. Fry tofu until golden brown.

4. Add noodles, sauce, carrots, green onions, and half of the cilantro to the pan with tofu. Stir until warmed through.

5. Serve immediately, topped with peanuts, remaining cilantro, and lime wedges. Optionally, serve with mung bean sprouts.

- For gluten-free, use tamari instead of soy sauce.
- To make it vegetarian, replace tofu with vegetables like bell peppers and broccoli.
- Use pre-cut julienne carrots to save time.

- Per serving:
- 500 calories,
- 68g carbohydrates,
- 17g protein,
- 19g fat,
- 8g saturated fat,
- 754 mg sodium,
- 585 mg potassium,
- 5g fiber,
- 16g sugar,
- 5571 IU Vitamin A,
- 13 mg Vitamin C,
- 111 mg Calcium,
- 3mg Iron.

3. *Sweet Potato and Black Bean Tacos*

Sweet Potato and Black Bean Tacos are a delightful fusion of flavors and textures that elevate taco night to a whole new level. Tender chunks of roasted sweet potatoes, seasoned to perfection with smoky spices, mingle harmoniously with hearty black beans, creating a satisfying and nutritious filling. Nestled in warm, soft tortillas, each bite offers a burst of savory goodness complemented by the natural sweetness of the sweet potatoes. Topped with a vibrant array of fresh toppings such as crunchy lettuce, creamy avocado slices, tangy salsa, and a drizzle of lime-infused crema, these tacos not only tantalize the taste buds but also provide a colorful feast for the eyes. Whether enjoyed as a quick weeknight dinner or a festive gathering with friends, Sweet Potato and Black Bean Tacos are sure to become a favorite, offering a deliciously wholesome twist on traditional taco flavors.

<u>*Preparetion Time:*</u>

- 10 minutes
- Cook Time:
- 30 minutes
- Total Time:
- 40 minutes
- Servings:
- 4 to 6 servings

<u>Ingredients</u>

For the roasted sweet potatoes:

- 1 to 2 medium sweet potatoes, cut into 1/2-inch cubes (about 2 cups)
- 2 tbsp neutral cooking oil (like grapeseed or canola)
- 1/2 tsp kosher salt
- 1 tsp chili powder
- 1/2 tsp ground cumin

For the beans:

- 2 tbsp neutral cooking oil (like grapeseed or canola)
- 1/2 medium yellow onion, diced (about 1/2 cup)
- 1/2 tsp kosher salt, plus more to taste
- 1 clove garlic, minced
- 1 jalapeño, seeded and minced
- 1 (15-ounce) can black beans, drained and rinsed
- Apple cider vinegar or water, as needed

To serve:

- 10 to 12 corn tortillas
- 1/2 cup tomatillo salsa verde (store-bought or homemade)
- 1 ripe avocado, thinly sliced
- Fresh cilantro, chopped
- Lime wedges
- 1/4 cup crumbled cotija cheese

1. Preheat your oven to 425°F (220°C).

2. Prepare the sweet potatoes:

- In a medium bowl, mix sweet potatoes with 2 tablespoons of oil, salt, cumin, and chili powder until coated.
- Spread evenly on a baking sheet. Bake for 30 minutes, flipping halfway, until tender and crispy.

3. Sweet Potato and Black Bean Tacos

4. Cook the black beans:

- While sweet potatoes bake, heat 2 tablespoons of oil in a medium saucepan over medium heat.
- Sauté onions with 1/2 teaspoon of salt until soft (5-7 minutes).
- Add garlic and jalapeño, sauté for 2 more minutes, then stir in black beans.
- Cook for 10-15 minutes, stirring occasionally, until beans are soft and

seasoned. Add a splash of apple cider vinegar or water if needed. Adjust salt to taste.

5. Prepare the tortillas:

- Warm tortillas in a dry skillet or microwave until heated through.

6. Assemble the tacos:

- Place sweet potatoes and black beans on each tortilla.
- Serve with avocado, salsa, cilantro, and cotija cheese for toppings.

Enjoy your Sweet Potato and Black Bean Tacos!

Nutritional Information

- (each portion)
- 434: Energy
- 23g: Fat Content
- 52g: Carbohydrates
- 11g:Protein

4.Vegan chili

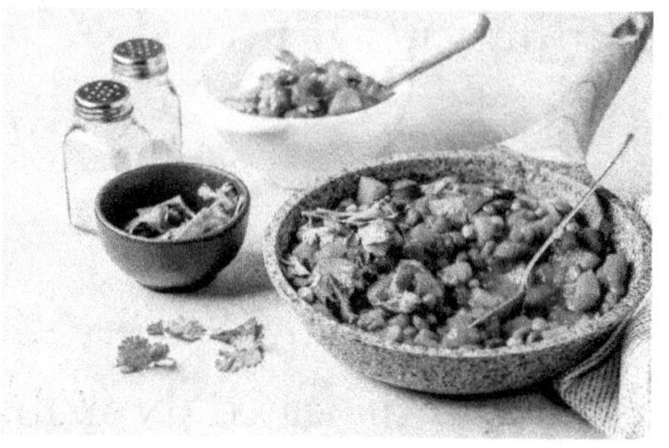

Vegan chili is a hearty dish made from plants. It has beans (like kidney, black, or chickpeas), veggies (like tomatoes, bell peppers, onions, and corn), and spices (like chili powder, cumin, paprika, and garlic). This stew is cooked slowly to blend flavors and make a tasty, nutritious meal. Great for cold nights or relaxed get-togethers, vegan chili has a mix of textures and flavors that everyone enjoys, whether they're vegan or not.

Preparation time:

- 10 minutes
- Cooking time:
- 30 minutes
- Total time:

- 40 minutes
- Servings: 6-8

Ingredients list:

1. 1 small yellow onion, diced
2. 2 green bell peppers, diced
3. 3 ribs celery, diced
4. 3 cloves garlic, minced
5. 3 small carrots, thinly sliced
6. 4 tablespoons ancho chili powder*
7. 1 tablespoon ground cumin
8. 1 teaspoon dried oregano
9. Optional: ½ teaspoon cayenne pepper
10. 1 teaspoon sea salt
11. 2 cans (15 ounces each) red kidney beans, drained
12. 2 cans (15 ounces each) pinto beans, drained
13. 2 cans (28 ounces each) crushed tomatoes
14. 1 cup (235 ml) low-sodium vegetable broth (or water)
15. Optional toppings: green onions, nutritional yeast, vegan sour cream

1. Heat a large pot over medium-high heat. Add 1/3 cup of water (or oil) and put in the onion, celery, and green pepper. Cook until the water evaporates, stirring occasionally. It should take about 10 minutes until the veggies turn golden brown. Add another 1/4 cup of water to loosen any bits stuck to the pot.

2. Reduce the heat to medium. Add garlic, carrots, chili powder, cumin, oregano, salt, and cayenne pepper (if using). Sauté for 2-3 minutes, adding a splash of water if things stick.

3. Add kidney beans, pinto beans, crushed tomatoes, and vegetable broth to the pot. Bring to a boil over high heat, then lower to a simmer. Cover and cook for 10 minutes. Uncover and cook for another 5-7 minutes until the carrots are tender and the chili thickens, stirring occasionally.

4. Serve hot, garnishing as desired. Store leftovers in an airtight container in the fridge for up to 5 days or freeze for up to one month. Reheat on the stove or in the microwave before serving.

Notes

1.Chili Powder: Use pure ancho chili powder for better flavor instead of blends with different spices and salt. If using a blend with salt, use only 1/2 teaspoon and adjust to taste.

2.Beans: You can swap pinto or kidney beans with black beans, or try my Chipotle Black Bean Chili recipe!

3.Cooking with Oil: Heat 1 tablespoon of oil and sauté onion, celery, and green pepper until they start sticking. Add 1/4 cup of water to deglaze the pan in step one, scraping the bottom as needed. Then continue with the recipe.

4. Meat Option: If you want a meaty chili, cook vegan "ground" or chopped sausage with garlic and spices in step 2.

Nutritional Information

- Calories:About 250 per cup
- Protein: Around 12 grams per serving
- Carbohydrates: About 45 grams, with 15 grams of fiber and 10 grams of sugars
- Fat: About 3 grams, with less than 1 gram of saturated fat
- Sodium: Around 800 mg (varies depending on what you put in)
- Vitamins and Minerals: Includes good amounts of vitamin A, vitamin C, iron, and potassium from beans, tomatoes, and veggies.

These amounts can change based on what ingredients you use and how you make your chili.

5. Cauliflower and Chickpea Shawarma Wraps

Enjoy our Cauliflower and Chickpea Shawarma Wraps, where roasted cauliflower and chickpeas with Middle Eastern spices are wrapped in a soft tortilla with lettuce, tomatoes, and tahini sauce. Each bite is a mix of textures and flavors for a satisfying meal, great for lunch or dinner.

Preparetion time:

- 15 minutes

Ingredients:

- 1 pound cauliflower, cut into small florets
- 1 (15.5 ounce) can chickpeas, drained and dried
- 1 teaspoon ground cumin
- 1 teaspoon garlic powder
- 1 teaspoon sweet paprika
- 1 teaspoon ground turmeric
- 1 teaspoon ground coriander

- 1/2 teaspoon sea salt
- 1/4 teaspoon ground cinnamon
- 1/4 teaspoon ground ginger
- 1/4 teaspoon black pepper
- 1/8 teaspoon cayenne pepper
- 1/4 cup olive oil
- Juice of half a lemon
- 2 whole wheat pitas or wraps

For the Yogurt Dill Sauce:
- 1 cup non-dairy plain yogurt
- Juice of half a lemon
- 2 cloves garlic, minced
- 1 tablespoon chopped fresh dill (or dried dill)
- 1 small cucumber, grated and squeezed to remove excess water
- Salt and pepper, to taste

<u>**Instructions**</u>

Step 1: Preheat the Oven

- Start by preheating your oven to 425ºF (about 220ºC). Line a baking sheet with parchment paper and set it aside.

Step 2: Prepare the Vegetables

- In a medium-sized bowl, combine the chickpeas and cauliflower. In another small bowl, mix together the spices, oil, and lemon juice until thoroughly blended. Pour this seasoning mixture over the vegetables and toss gently to ensure even coating.

Step 3: Roast in the Oven

- Spread the seasoned chickpeas and cauliflower evenly on the prepared baking sheet. Place it in the preheated oven and roast for 25-30 minutes. Remember to flip and rotate the vegetables halfway through the cooking time to achieve uniform crispiness.

Step 4: Prepare the Tzatziki Sauce

- While the vegetables are roasting, prepare the tzatziki sauce. Combine all the sauce ingredients in a bowl, mixing well until smooth and creamy.

Step 5: Assemble and Serve

- Warm the pita bread briefly. To assemble each wrap, spoon a generous amount of the roasted chickpeas and cauliflower onto the center of a pita. Drizzle with tzatziki sauce according to taste.

- Optionally, add fresh garnishes like lettuce, diced tomatoes, or red onions for added flavor and texture.

- Roll up the pita and serve immediately, ensuring all the delicious flavors are enjoyed together.

This method offers a delightful blend of roasted chickpeas and cauliflower wrapped in warm pita bread, enhanced by the refreshing tang of homemade tzatziki sauce.

Nutritional Value (Per Serving):

- Calories : About 350-400
- Protein : 12-15 grams
- Carbohydrates : 50-55 grams
- Fiber : 8-10 grams
- Sugar : 5-8 grams
- Fat : 12-15 grams
- Saturated Fat : 1-2 grams
- Sodium : 500-600 mg (varies with seasoning and tzatziki)
- Potassium: 400-500 mg
- Vitamin C: Provides 40-50% of your daily needs
- Iron: Provides 15-20% of your daily needs
- Calcium: Provides 10-15% of your daily needs

- Cauliflower and chickpeas for protein and fiber
- Pita bread for carbohydrates
- Spices (cumin, paprika, garlic powder)
- Olive oil and lemon juice for flavor and healthy fats
- Tzatziki sauce (yogurt, cucumber, garlic, dill, lemon juice) for creaminess and tang
- Optional garnishes like lettuce, tomato, and red onion for extra flavor and texture

Summary:

Cauliflower and Chickpea Shawarma Wraps provide a balanced mix of protein, carbohydrates, healthy fats, and essential vitamins and minerals like Vitamin C and Iron. They're nutritious and filling, perfect for a satisfying meal.

6. Grilled Portobello Mushrooms

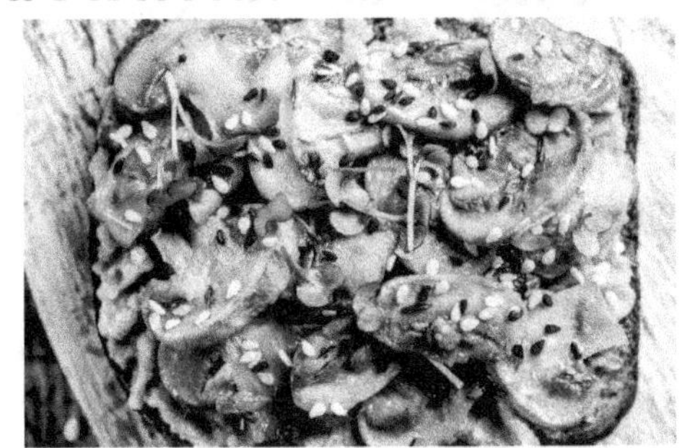

Grilled Portobello Mushrooms are delicious and packed with flavor, appealing to both vegetarians and meat lovers. Each mushroom cap is grilled perfectly to give it a smoky smell and enhance its rich, savory taste. They're great on their own or added to salads, sandwiches, or pasta for a tasty and satisfying meal.

To make delicious marinated grilled mushrooms, begin with hearty portobello mushrooms. Gather a few common ingredients to make a tasty marinade that enhances the mushrooms' natural earthy flavor when you grill them.

Preparation time:

- 10 minutes
- Cook time:
- 6 minutes
- Total time:
- 25 minutes
- Servings: 4

Ingredients:

- 4 large portobello mushrooms, stems and gills removed, wiped clean
- ¼ cup balsamic vinegar
- 1 tablespoon extra virgin olive oil
- 1 tablespoon low sodium soy sauce
- 1 tablespoon chopped fresh rosemary (or 1/2 teaspoon dried rosemary)
- 1 teaspoon garlic powder
- ½ teaspoon black pepper
- ⅛ teaspoon cayenne pepper (optional, adjust to taste)
- Canola or vegetable oil for grilling

<u>***Optional for serving:***</u>

- Herby Avocado Sauce
- Burger buns
- Cheese (optional)
- Fresh toppings like spinach, tomato, avocado

<u>*Instructions:*</u>

1. Mix balsamic vinegar, olive oil, soy sauce, rosemary, garlic powder, black pepper, and cayenne pepper in a shallow dish. Add mushrooms, turning to coat evenly. Let them marinate for at least 5 minutes on each side, or up to 30 minutes for stronger flavor.

2. Heat your grill or skillet to medium (350 to 400°F). Lightly brush with oil to prevent sticking.

3. Remove mushrooms from marinade, shaking off excess liquid. Save the marinade for basting.

4. Grill mushrooms for 3-4 minutes on each side until caramelized and golden brown. Brush with reserved marinade during cooking.

5. Serve grilled portobello mushrooms topped with Herby Avocado Sauce or preferred toppings. They can also be served as burgers with buns, cheese, spinach, tomato, and avocado.

Additional Tips:

- Ensure your grill or skillet is hot enough for good searing.
- Use a grill pan indoors if preferred.
- Avoid crowding mushrooms in the skillet for even cooking.
- Try different toppings to customize flavors.
- Leftovers can be refrigerated and reheated gently.

<u>*Tips*</u>

Freshly grilled mushrooms taste best but can be kept in the fridge for a few days. Use leftovers by chopping them and adding to scrambled eggs for a healthy lunch.

<u>Nutritional fact</u>

- Serving Size: 1 out of 4 servings
- Calories: 60 kcal
- Carbohydrates: 9 grams
- Protein: 3 grams
- Fat: 2 grams
- Fiber: 1 gram
- Sugar: 7 grams

<u>**Note:**</u> The nutrition values are estimated based on using half of the marinade, which is mostly thrown away. These estimates are provided in good faith. For personalized adjustments, visit myfitnesspal.com.

7. Mango Quinoa Salad

Mango Quinoa Salad is a bright and tasty dish that mixes nutty quinoa with sweet, juicy mangoes. It also includes crunchy bell peppers, red onions, and fresh cilantro, all dressed in a tangy lime sauce. This salad is a light and healthy choice that's full of different textures and flavors.

How to Slice a Mango (two simple methods)

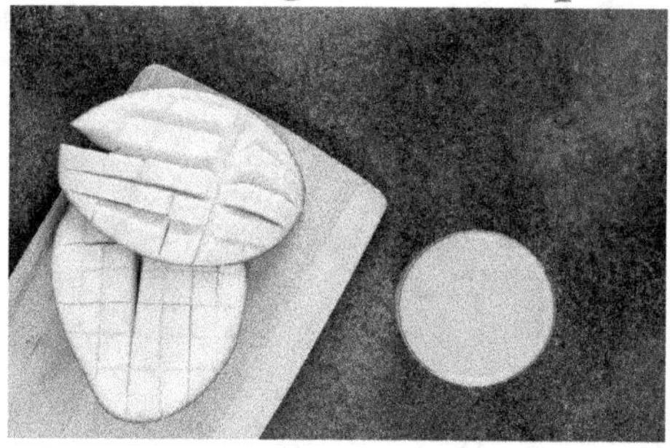

<u>*Preparetion Time:*</u>

- 5 minutes
- Total Time:
- 5 minutes
- Servings: 2

- Calories: 50 kcal

Equipment:
- Chef's Knife
- Paring Knife
- Pint Glass

Ingredients:
- 1 ripe mango

Instructions:

1. Cut the Mango:
   - Slice off the two large sides of the mango, avoiding the pit in the middle.

2. Peel with a Pint Glass:
   - Place one mango half upright on the rim of a pint glass. Press down gently to peel the mango away from the flesh.

3. Dice the Mango:

- Score the mango flesh with a knife to make a grid pattern, but don't cut through the skin. Flip the mango to separate the cubes a bit.
- Use a small knife to cut the cubes off the skin.

4. Cut Remaining Mango:
- Slice off the remaining mango flesh around the pit.
- Peel the strips and cut them into small cubes.

Notes:

- A small to medium mango usually gives about 1 cup of diced fruit, but larger ones can provide up to 2 cups.
- Use the diced mango in yogurt, smoothies, or recipes like Mango Quinoa Salad or Mango Salsa.

<u>**Nutrition Information (per serving):**</u>

- Calories: 50 kcal
- Carbohydrates: 12g
- Protein: 1g
- Fat: 1g
- Saturated Fat: 1g
- Sodium: 1mg
- Potassium: 139 mg
- Fiber: 1g
- Sugar: 11g
- Vitamin A: 893 IU
- Vitamin C: 30mg
- Calcium: 9mg
- Iron: 1mg

<u>*Chilled Mango Quinoa Salad*</u>

<u>*Preparation Time:*</u>

- 5 minutes
- Cooking Time:
- 15 minutes
- Total Time:

- 20 minutes.
- Servings: 4. Calories per serving: 249 kcal.

Ingredients:

- 1/2 cup uncooked quinoa
- 1 large diced mango (about 1 cup)
- 1 pint halved cherry tomatoes
- 1/4 cup finely chopped red onion
- 1 jalapeño, seeded and finely chopped
- 1/4 cup chopped fresh cilantro
- Juice and zest of 1 lime
- 1/4 cup extra-virgin olive oil
- Salt and black pepper, to taste

Instructions:

1. Rinse quinoa until water runs clear. Cook in a pot with 1 cup water and a pinch of salt. Boil, cover, and simmer for 15 minutes. Let it sit covered for 5 minutes.

2. Mix lime zest, lime juice, olive oil, salt, and pepper in a large bowl.

3. Rinse cooked quinoa with cold water and drain well.

4. Add the quinoa, mango, tomatoes, jalapeño, and onion to the bowl with the dressing. Toss to mix.

5. Chill in the fridge for at least an hour before serving.

- For a more filling meal, add black beans, chickpeas, chicken, or steak.
- Prepare other ingredients while the quinoa cooks to save time.

Nutrition Information (per serving):

- Calories: 249
- Carbs: 26g
- Protein: 5g
- Fat: 15g
- Saturated Fat: 2g
- Sodium: 16mg
- Potassium: 473mg
- Fiber: 3g

- Sugar: 9g
- Vitamin A: 1126IU
- Vitamin C: 48mg
- Calcium: 28mg
- Iron: 2mg

8. Millet-Stuffed Bell Peppers

Millet-Stuffed Bell Peppers are a healthy and tasty meal where colorful bell peppers are filled with a mixture of cooked millet, veggies, and spices. The millet is cooked until soft and mixed with onions, garlic, tomatoes, and herbs. This mixture is seasoned well and used to stuff each bell pepper. The peppers are then baked until soft and topped with fresh herbs. This dish is a great plant-based option that brings out the sweet flavor of the peppers.

Preparation time:

- 20 minutes
- Cook time:
- 40 minutes
- Total time:
- 1 hour
- Serves: 4 people

Ingredients:

- 4 bell peppers of any color
- 1 cup cooked millet
- 1 onion, diced
- 2 garlic cloves, minced
- 1 zucchini, diced
- 1 tomato, diced
- 1 tsp cumin
- 1 tsp ground coriander
- Salt and black pepper, to taste

Instructions:

1. Preheat your oven to 375°F.

2. Slice off the tops of the bell peppers and remove the seeds and membranes inside.

3. Heat a pan and sauté the diced onion and minced garlic until they become translucent.

4. Add the diced zucchini, tomato, and spices to the pan. Cook until the vegetables are tender.

5. Mix in the cooked millet and stir for a few more minutes.

6. Fill each bell pepper with the millet and vegetable mixture. Stand the peppers upright in a baking dish.

7. Cover the dish with aluminum foil and bake for 35 minutes.

8. Remove the foil and bake for an additional 5 minutes.

9. Serve while hot.

Nutrition Information (per serving):

- Calories: 171 kcal
- Total Fat: 1 g
- Saturated Fat: 0 g
- Cholesterol: 0 mg
- Sodium: 63 mg
- Total Carbohydrates: 38 g
- Dietary Fiber: 9 g
- Sugars: 13 g
- Protein: 7 g

9. Jackfruit Tacos

Jackfruit tacos are a fun twist on regular tacos. The jackfruit has a meaty texture and soaks up spices and herbs when cooked, giving it a rich and slightly sweet taste. These tacos are often topped with crunchy cabbage, tangy lime sauce, and flavorful salsa, and can be served in soft or crunchy tortillas. They make a tasty and filling plant-based meal with lots of different flavors and textures.

Ingredients

- For the Jackfruit:
- 2 cans (20 oz each) green jackfruit in water or brine, drained, rinsed, and chopped
- 1 tablespoon oil (like canola or vegetable)
- 1 yellow onion, sliced
- 4 cloves garlic, minced
- ½ cup vegetable broth or water
- 1 tablespoon agave syrup
- Juice from ½ lime

- 2 teaspoons chili powder
- 1 teaspoon cumin
- 1 teaspoon smoked paprika
- ¼ teaspoon salt

For the Tacos:

- 8 taco shells (hard or soft, gluten-free if preferred)
- 1 avocado, sliced
- ¼ red onion, sliced
- ¼ cup chopped cilantro
- Lime wedges

Instructions

Preparing the Jackfruit:

Cut the jackfruit into thin slices from the core to the outside. This helps make it shred better. Don't throw away the core or seeds—they're edible!

Heat oil in a large pan over medium-high heat. Add chopped onions and garlic, cooking for about 5 minutes until the onions are soft and a little brown.

Add the jackfruit, broth, agave syrup, lime juice, and spices to the pan. Cover and simmer on low heat until the jackfruit is soft and half of the liquid is absorbed, about 5 minutes.

Mash the jackfruit with a potato masher to shred it. If it's too wet, cook longer. If it's too dry, add a little more broth.

Assembling the Tacos:

Warm the taco shells according to the package instructions. Fill each shell with the shredded jackfruit, then add avocado slices, red onion slices, cilantro, and a squeeze of lime juice. Add any other favorite taco toppings or a bit of hot sauce if you like.

Nutritional value

- Calories : 265
- Carbs : 49 grams
- Protein : 2 grams
- Fat : 8 grams
- Saturated Fat : 1 gram
- Salt : 188 milligrams
- Potassium: 337 milligrams
- Fiber : 5 grams
- Sugar : 3 grams
- Vitamin A: 373 IU
- Vitamin C: 6 milligrams
- Calcium: 88 milligrams
- Iron : 1 milligram

10. Curried Cauliflower and Chickpea

Curried Cauliflower and Chickpeas is a tasty and filling meal with soft cauliflower and protein-packed chickpeas cooked in a spicy curry sauce. It usually includes spices like cumin, coriander, turmeric, and garam masala that give the vegetables a warm, rich taste. Often topped with fresh herbs like cilantro and a splash of lemon or coconut milk, this dish is a comforting, creamy, and healthy vegetarian choice.

Ingredients

- 4 cups cauliflower florets
- 2 tablespoons olive oil
- Salt and pepper
- Garlic powder
- 1 sweet onion, chopped
- 4 garlic cloves, minced
- 3 tablespoons fresh ginger, minced
- 1 ½ tablespoons curry powder (more if you like)
- 1 teaspoon ground turmeric

- 2 (14-ounce) cans chickpeas, rinsed and drained
- 1 (14-ounce) can coconut milk
- ½ cup vegetable or chicken broth
- 2 tablespoons lime juice
- 2 green onions, sliced
- ½ cup chopped fresh cilantro
- Jasmine rice, for serving
- Naan bread, for serving

Instructions

1. Roast Cauliflower: Heat oven to 425°F (220°C). Place cauliflower on a baking sheet, drizzle with olive oil, and season with salt, pepper, and garlic powder. Roast for 20-25 minutes until tender and golden.

2. Prepare the Base: While cauliflower roasts, heat a tablespoon of olive oil in a large pot over medium-low heat. Add chopped onion, minced garlic, and a pinch of salt and pepper. Cook until onions are soft, about 5 minutes. Add minced ginger and cook for another minute.

3. Add Spices: Stir in curry powder and turmeric. Cook for 5 minutes until the spices are fragrant.

4. Combine Ingredients: Pour in the coconut milk and broth. Add chickpeas and roasted cauliflower. Stir in lime juice. Bring to a boil, then lower the heat and simmer for 5-10 minutes.

5. Finish and Serve: Taste and adjust seasoning if needed. Top with green onions and cilantro. Serve with jasmine rice and naan bread.

Nutritional Information (per serving, for 4 servings)

- Calories: About 430
- Protein: 14 grams
- Fat: 26 grams
- Carbohydrates : 43 grams

- Fiber : 10 grams
- Sugar : 8 grams
- Sodium : 700 mg

This is an estimate and can vary based on ingredient brands and portion sizes.

Chapter 5: Snacks and Appetizers

Chapter 5 of this cookbook is packed with easy and tasty snacks and appetizers that are perfect for any event. This section offers a wide range of options, from simple finger foods to delicious dips. Whether you're hosting a casual hangout with friends or a special occasion, the recipes here are designed to help you make enjoyable and impressive snacks.

You'll find clear, step-by-step instructions for a variety of treats that are both easy to make and satisfying. The chapter includes classic favorites and some unique ideas that are sure to add excitement to your menu. Whether it's simple appetizers or more elaborate dips, the recipes are straightforward and great for cooks of all skill levels.

This chapter provides plenty of ideas to make any gathering special, with recipes that accommodate different tastes and dietary needs. You'll also get tips on how to present your snacks in an appealing way.

In summary, Chapter 5 is your guide to creating a fantastic spread of snacks and appetizers. No matter the size or type of your event, these recipes will help ensure your guests have a great time and enjoy memorable food.

1. Raw Vegetables with Hummus

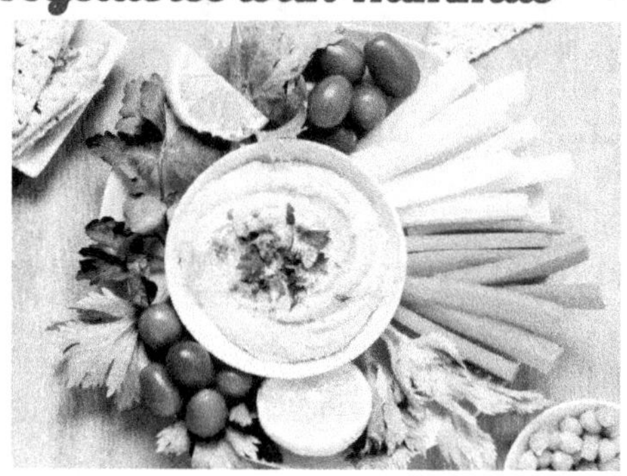

Raw vegetables with hummus is a tasty and healthy snack. You get fresh, crunchy veggies like carrots, celery, bell peppers, cucumbers, and cherry tomatoes. They're paired with hummus, which is a smooth mix of chickpeas, tahini, lemon juice, and garlic. This snack is good for you because it has fiber, protein, and healthy fats. It's a great choice for a quick, nutritious bite.

Preparation Time:

- 10 minutes

Ingredients:

- 1 cup carrot sticks
- 1 cup cucumber slices
- 1 cup bell pepper strips
- 1/2 cup plain or lemon-flavored hummus

Instructions:

1. Wash and cut the vegetables into sticks or slices.
2. Arrange the vegetables on a plate and serve with hummus on the side.

Nutritional Value (per 1 cup of vegetables with 2 tbsp hummus):

- Calories: ~100
- Carbohydrates: 14g
- Protein: 4g
- Fiber: 4g

 Use a low-sodium hummus to minimize added salt. You can also vary the vegetables based on your preferences and seasonal availability.

2.Cucumber and Avocado Slices

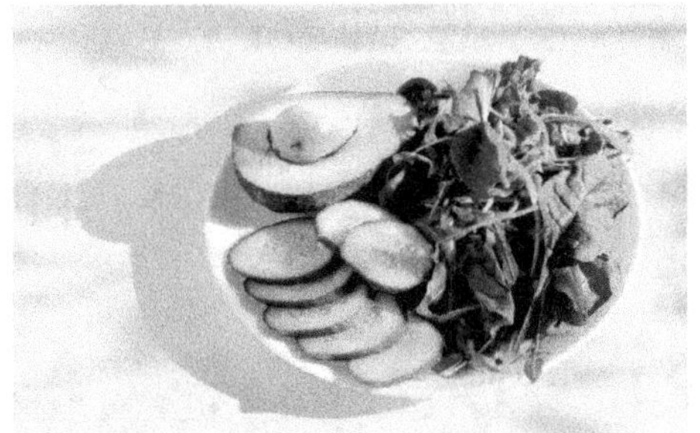

Cucumber and avocado slices are a tasty, healthy snack. The cucumbers are crunchy, and the avocados are smooth and creamy. This simple snack is great for a light bite or as an appetizer.

Preparation Time:

- 10 minutes

Ingredients:

Serves 4 as a side salad

- 2 English cucumbers, sliced thinly
- 1 large avocado, peeled, pitted, and sliced
- 1/3 cup chopped green onions (approximately half a bunch)
- 2 tablespoons lime juice (from 1 medium lime)

- 2 tablespoons extra virgin olive oil
- 1 teaspoon sea salt (or 3/4 teaspoon table salt, to taste)
- 1/8 teaspoon ground black pepper

<u>*Nutritional Value (per serving, about 1 cup):*</u>

- Calories: 120
- Protein: 2 g
- Carbohydrates:12 g
- Fat: 9 g
- Fiber: 6 g
- Vitamin C:10% DV
- Vitamin K: 20% DV
- Potassium: 400 mg

<u>*Instructions:*</u>

1.Prepare Ingredients: Wash the cucumber and cut it into thin rounds. Cut the avocado in half, remove the pit, and slice it thinly.

2. Assemble: Place the cucumber slices on a plate and put a piece of avocado on each one.

3. Season (Optional): Add a little salt, pepper, or lemon juice if you like.

4. Serve: Eat right away for the best taste and texture.

Tips:

- Use a ripe avocado for a creamy feel. Let it ripen if it's too firm.
- To stop the avocado from browning, eat it soon or brush with lemon juice.
- Add fresh herbs like dill or cilantro for extra flavor if you want.

3. Rice Cakes with Avocado

Rice cakes with avocado make a tasty and light snack or meal. The crunchy rice cakes are great with smooth avocado spread on top. Just spread some ripe avocado on the rice cake, add a little salt and pepper, and maybe some red pepper flakes or lemon juice for extra flavor. This snack is both yummy and good for you, full of healthy fats and nutrients.

<u>Preparation Time:</u>

- 5 minutes

Ingredients:

- 2 plain rice cakes
- 1 ripe avocado
- A pinch of salt (optional)
- A squeeze of lemon juice (optional)

Instructions:

1. Mash the avocado in a bowl.
2. Spread the mashed avocado evenly over the rice cakes.
3. Season with a pinch of salt and a squeeze of lemon juice if desired.

<u>Nutritional Value (per serving of 2 rice cakes with avocado):</u>

- Calories: ~150
- Carbohydrates: 15g
- Protein: 2g

- Fat: 10g (mostly healthy fats from avocado)

Tips: Choose rice cakes that are free from added sugars or preservatives. For extra flavor, you can add a sprinkle of herbs or spices.

4. Chia Seed Pudding

Chia seed pudding is a smooth, healthy treat made by soaking chia seeds in a liquid like almond milk, coconut milk, or regular milk. Adding a sweetener like honey or maple syrup and flavors such as vanilla or cocoa powder makes the seeds expand and turn into a jelly-like consistency. You can enjoy it on its own or add fruits, nuts, or granola for extra taste and crunch. It's a great, filling choice that's full of fiber and omega-3s and can be eaten anytime.

Preparation Time:

- 15 minutes
- Chilling Time:
- 8 hours

- Total Time:
- 8 hours 15 minutes
- Serves 1

Equipment
- Weck Mini Tulip Jars

Ingredients:
- ½ cup unsweetened almond milk
- 2 tablespoons chia seeds
- ½ teaspoon maple syrup
- ⅛ teaspoon cinnamon

Optional Toppings:
- Tart cherries
- Blueberries
- Nuts or granola
- Coconut flakes
- More maple syrup

Instructions:

1. In a jar with a lid, mix almond milk, chia seeds, maple syrup, and cinnamon.

2. Shake the jar thoroughly, then refrigerate for a few hours.

3. Stir the mixture to break up any clumps.

4. Let it sit in the fridge for 8 hours or overnight to thicken.

5. When ready to serve, add your preferred toppings like fruit, nuts, coconut flakes, or extra maple syrup.

Nutritional Value (per 1/2 cup serving):

- Calories: ~150
- Carbohydrates: 15g
- Protein: 4g
- Fat: 7g

Tips: For added flavor or texture, mix in fresh fruit or a sprinkle of cinnamon before serving.

5. Oatmeal Energy Balls

Oatmeal Energy Balls are a healthy and easy snack. Just mix rolled oats with nut butter, honey, and extras like chocolate chips or dried fruit. Roll into balls and chill in the fridge. They give you a quick energy boost and are great for a quick snack.

Ingredients list:

- 1 1/2 cups of traditional rolled oats
- 1/2 cup of pure nut spread (such as peanut, almond, or cashew)
- 1/3 cup of honey or pure maple syrup
- 1/4 cup of chocolate morsels

Instructions

1. Mix Ingredients: In a large bowl, mix rolled oats, nut butter, honey, and chocolate chips until everything is well combined.

2. Chill: Put the bowl in the fridge for 15-20 minutes to make the mixture easier to shape.

3.Form Balls: After chilling, use a spoon or cookie scoop to scoop out the mixture and roll it into small balls with your hands.

4. Store: Keep the energy balls in an airtight container in the fridge. They stay fresh for up to a week.

Additional Tips :

- **Customize:** Add extras like shredded coconut, chia seeds, or dried fruit to change the flavor and add more nutrition.

- **Adjust Texture:** If the mixture is too sticky, add more oats. If it's too dry, add a bit more honey or nut butter.

- **Enjoy:** These energy balls are a great, quick snack, perfect for on-the-go or after exercise.

Tips:

- Dampen your hands a little to keep the mixture from sticking.
- Use a cookie scoop to make sure each ball is the same size.
- Press the mixture firmly when rolling to keep the balls from falling apart.

Nutrition:

Makes 15 servings

Serving Size: 1 ball

Each Serving: 105 calories, 5g total fat, 1g saturated fat, 0g trans fat, 3g unsaturated fat, 2mg cholesterol, 20mg sodium, 15g carbs, 1g fiber, 9g sugar, 2g protein

6. Banana and Nut Butter Snack

This quick and easy snack pairs sweet bananas with creamy nut butter. It's a tasty and nutritious option that's good for a vegan diet and gentle on migraines.

Preparation Time:
- 5 minutes

Ingredients:
- 1 ripe banana
- 2 tablespoons almond butter or other nut butter (pure and without additives)

Instructions

1. Slice the Banana: Peel the banana and cut it into thin rounds.

2. Add Nut Butter: Spread a little nut butter on each banana slice.

3. Arrange: Place the banana slices on a plate with the nut butter side up.

4. _Enjoy:_ Eat right away or chill in the fridge for a cold snack.

Nutritional Value (for 1 banana and 2 tablespoons of almond butter):

- Calories : About 250
- Protein : 6 grams
- Fat: 16 grams (mainly healthy fats)
- Carbs : 30 grams
- Fiber : 4 grams
- Sugar: 14 grams (from the banana)

Tips :

- Choose Simple Nut Butter: Pick nut butter with just nuts and a bit of salt.
- Try Different Nuts: Use other nut butters like cashew or peanut if they don't trigger your migraines.
- Watch Portions: Nut butter is calorie-rich, so use it in moderation.
- Add Flavor: Sprinkle a bit of cinnamon or chia seeds for extra taste.

This snack is quick, healthy, and easy to make, perfect for a busy day or a quick energy boost.

7. Avocado and Cucumber Sushi Rolls

Avocado and cucumber sushi rolls are a tasty and colorful twist on regular sushi. They have creamy avocado and crunchy cucumber wrapped in rice and seaweed. The avocado is smooth and rich, while the cucumber is crisp and cool. These rolls might be topped with sesame seeds or pickled ginger. They look great and are light and satisfying, making them a great choice for sushi fans and vegetarians.

Preparation time:

- Cooking time:
- 30 minutes
- Overall time:
- 45 minutes

Ingredients:

- 1 cup sushi rice
- 1 ¼ cup water

- 1 tbsp rice vinegar
- 1 tbsp maple syrup
- 1 large avocado, sliced
- 1 cucumber, cut into thin strips
- Nori sheets

Instructions:

1. Rinse rice until water is clear.

2. Cook rice with water according to rice cooker instructions.

3. Mix rice vinegar and maple syrup into the cooked rice.

4. Spread rice on a nori sheet, add avocado and cucumber, then roll tightly.

5. Slice into pieces.

Nutritional Info (2 rolls):

- Calories: ~140
- Protein: 2g
- Fat: 5g
- Carbs: 22g
- Fiber: 2g

Tips:
- Let rice cool before rolling.
- Use a sharp knife for clean slices.

8. Roasted Red Pepper Hummus

Roasted Red Pepper Hummus is a tasty and colorful take on the traditional Middle Eastern dip. It mixes creamy chickpeas with the sweet, smoky flavor of roasted red peppers, plus a touch of garlic, tahini, lemon juice, and olive oil. This hummus has a rich taste and looks great, making it ideal for dipping with pita bread, fresh veggies, or spreading on sandwiches and wraps.

Ingredients:

- 1 can chickpeas
- 1 roasted red bell pepper
- 2 tbsp tahini
- 2 tbsp lemon juice
- 1 garlic clove
- ¼ cup water
- Salt and pepper

Instructions:

1. Blend chickpeas, red pepper, tahini, lemon juice, and garlic in a food processor.

2. Add water to reach desired consistency.

3. Season with salt and pepper. Serve with veggies or crackers.

Nutritional Info (1/4 cup):

- Calories: ~100
- Protein: 4g
- Fat: 6g
- Carbs: 9g
- Fiber: 3g

Tips:

- Blend longer for creamier hummus.
- Store in the fridge for up to a week.

9. Stuffed Cherry Tomatoes

Stuffed Cherry Tomatoes are a tasty and fancy snack or side dish. Small tomatoes are scooped out and filled with a creamy mix, usually made with cream cheese or goat cheese, fresh herbs like basil or parsley, and a bit of garlic or onion. Sometimes, the filling is topped with breadcrumbs or nuts for extra crunch. The stuffed tomatoes are baked until the cheese is soft and the tomatoes are cooked but still firm. They have a fresh, tangy taste with creamy filling, making them a great choice for parties or as a tasty addition to any meal.

Preparation Time:

- 45 minutes
- Overall Time:
- 45 minutes

Ingredients:

- 20 cherry tomatoes
- 1 cup cooked quinoa
- ¼ cup chopped basil

- 2 tbsp nutritional yeast
- 1 tbsp lemon juice
- Salt and pepper

Instructions:

1. Cut tops off tomatoes and scoop out the insides.
2. Mix quinoa, basil, nutritional yeast, and lemon juice.
3. Season, then fill tomatoes with the mixture.

Nutritional Info (4 tomatoes):

- Calories: ~80
- Protein: 3g
- Fat: 2g
- Carbs: 12g
- Fiber: 2g

Tips:

- Add chopped peppers or cucumbers for extra flavor.
- Serve right away for the best taste.

10. Sweet Potato and Black Bean

"Sweet Potato and Black beans" is a short story about a unique dish. It takes place in a charming small town and follows Oliver, a quiet chef with a small restaurant known for its special dishes. One day, Oliver finds an old family recipe called "Sweet Potato and Black," which mixes sweet potatoes with black truffle and black beans.

As Oliver tries out this new recipe, he not only changes his restaurant's menu but also reconnects with old friends and family members who each have their own memories of the dish. Through this journey, Oliver learns more about his family's history and traditions. The story shows how food can help people reconnect and start fresh, celebrating both flavor and personal history.

Ingredients:

- 1 large sweet potato, diced
- 1 can black beans
- ½ tsp cumin

- ½ tsp paprika
- ¼ cup chopped cilantro
- Salt

Instructions:

1. Roast sweet potato cubes at 400°F (200°C) for 20 minutes.
2. Mix with black beans, cumin, paprika, and cilantro. Mash lightly.
3. Form into small balls and bake for 10 more minutes.

Nutritional Info (4 bites):

- Calories: ~120
- Protein: 4g
- Fat: 2g
- Carbs: 22g
- Fiber: 5g

Tips:

- Cook sweet potatoes well for easy mashing.
- Adjust spices to taste.

11. Crispy Chickpea Snacks

Crispy Chickpea Snacks are tasty, crunchy bites made from roasted chickpeas. They're seasoned with spices for a savory flavor in every crunch. These snacks are great for a healthy option or as a crunchy addition to salads and soups. They're high in protein and low in fat, making them a better choice than many other snacks. Enjoy them anytime or share with friends for a healthy treat.

Ingredients:

- 1 can chickpeas
- 1 tbsp olive oil
- 1 tsp paprika
- 1 tsp garlic powder
- Salt

Instructions:

1. Toss chickpeas with oil, paprika, garlic powder, and salt.
2. Bake at 400°F (200°C) for 20-25 minutes, shaking pan occasionally.

3. Cool before serving.

Nutritional Info (¼ cup):

- Calories: ~130
- Protein: 6g
- Fat: 5g
- Carbs: 18g
- Fiber: 5g

Tips:

- Dry chickpeas thoroughly before baking for crispiness.
- Try different spices for variety.

Conclusion

In this chapter, we've covered a variety of snacks and appetizers that are sure to please everyone and fit any occasion. From classic dips to easy finger foods, these recipes are tasty and simple. Perfecting these appetizers will help you create memorable gatherings and enjoyable snacks.

In the next chapter, we'll move on to desserts and treats. You'll find ideas for sweet treats, from rich cakes to light and refreshing options. Whether you want to end a meal on a high note or enjoy a sweet snack, the next chapter will show you the best desserts.

Chapter 6: Desserts and Treats

Step into a realm of sweetness with Chapter 6, where indulgence and pleasure shine. This chapter is dedicated to an array of desserts and treats, featuring recipes that span from timeless classics to creative new ideas. You'll discover comprehensive instructions for baking moist cakes, crafting delicate pastries, and whipping up rich, satisfying puddings. Each recipe is crafted to be both accessible and impressive, complete with tips to refine your skills and enhance your presentations. Whether you're seeking a simple yet sophisticated dessert or something to impress a gathering, this chapter provides everything you need to end your meals on a perfect note.

6.1 Decadent Vegan Desserts

1.Pear and Almond Crisp

A Pear and Almond Crisp is a yummy dessert made with soft, sweet pears covered by a crunchy, buttery topping. The pears are mixed with a little sugar and spices, then topped with a mix of oats, almond flour, and brown sugar. When baked, it turns golden brown and gives a sweet, nutty taste with a nice crunch. It's perfect for a cozy night in.

Preparation time:

- 15 minutes
- Cooking time:
- 40-45 minutes

Ingredients

- About 3 pounds Bosc or Anjou pears, peeled and cored
- 1 tablespoon brown sugar
- 1 tablespoon lemon juice

- Zest from 1 lemon

- 3/4 cup all-purpose flour
- 1 cup light brown sugar
- 1/2 teaspoon salt
- 1/2 teaspoon ground cinnamon
- 1/2 teaspoon ground dried ginger
- 1/4 teaspoon ground nutmeg
- 1 stick (8 tablespoons) unsalted butter, cubed, plus 1 tablespoon for greasing
- 1 cup Fisher Slivered Almonds, chopped

Instructions

1. Preheat the oven to 375°F.

2. Pears: Cut the pears into thin slices after removing the core and halving. Combine them in a large bowl with brown sugar, lemon juice, and zest. Set aside.

3. Topping: In a medium bowl, blend flour, brown sugar, salt, cinnamon, ginger, and nutmeg. Mix in the butter and almonds with your fingers until the mixture is crumbly.

4. Grease an 8-inch square baking dish with the remaining butter. Layer the pears in the dish and evenly distribute the topping over them. Bake in the center of the oven for 40-45 minutes, or until the pears are soft and the topping is golden brown. Allow to cool slightly before serving.

Nutritional value per serving (estimate):

- Calories: 350
- Total fat: 16g
- Saturated fat: 8g
- Cholesterol: 30mg
- Sodium: 150mg
- Total carbohydrates: 50g
- Dietary fiber: 4g
- Sugars: 35g
- Protein: 3g
- Guilt-Free Sweet Snacks

2. Raw Carrot Cake

Raw carrot cake is a tasty and healthy version of traditional carrot cake that doesn't need baking. It's made with grated carrots, nuts, seeds, and spices, sweetened with dates or maple syrup. Sometimes, coconut, raisins, or apples are added for extra flavor and texture. The mix is pressed into a pan and chilled until it's firm. It's a nutritious way to enjoy the classic carrot cake flavor.

Ingredients

Carrot Cake:

- 2 cups walnuts
- 2 cups pitted Medjool dates
- 1 cup unsweetened shredded coconut
- Juice and zest of 1/2 lemon
- 2 tsp vanilla extract
- 2 tsp ground cinnamon
- 1 tsp ground ginger
- 1/4 tsp ground nutmeg

- 1/2 cup coconut flour
- 2 cups finely grated carrots

Carrot Cake Frosting:
- 2 cups soaked cashews
- 1/2 cup coconut cream
- 1/4 cup melted coconut oil
- 1/4 cup plus 1 Tbsp maple syrup
- 1/4 cup lemon juice
- 1 tsp vanilla extract

Equipment:
- Food processor
- Blender
- Springform pan
- Strainer
- Can opener
- Liquid measuring cup
- Measuring cups and spoons

To make the carrot cake, start by grinding the walnuts in a food processor until they are finely chopped but still a bit chunky. Add dates, shredded coconut, lemon juice, lemon zest, vanilla extract, and spices, and blend until it starts to stick together. Mix in the coconut flour and grated carrots with a spatula.

Press this mixture into a 6-inch springform pan, smoothing it out evenly. Freeze it for 10-15 minutes to set. If you only have one pan, freeze the first layer, then transfer it to a cake board and clean the pan before making the second layer.

For the frosting, blend cashews, coconut milk, coconut oil, maple syrup, lemon juice, and vanilla extract until smooth. Spread half of the frosting on the first cake layer and freeze for about 30 minutes. Add the second cake layer on top, pressing it down gently, and then spread the rest of the frosting on top.

Wrap the pan tightly with plastic wrap and a paper towel to prevent moisture, and freeze for at least 6 hours or overnight. When ready to eat, take the cake out of the pan. Serve it frozen or let it thaw for 15-20 minutes. Store leftovers in the refrigerator for up to a week or freeze for up to a month.

Notes:

- Use finely shredded coconut for a smoother cake.
- Squeeze extra moisture from the carrots to keep the cake light.
- Soak cashews in water for at least 8 hours to make them easier to blend. Adding a bit of salt can help too.
- For a raw version, use raw coconut cream from fresh coconuts.
- Prep time does not include soaking cashews and chilling the coconut milk.

<u>***Nutrition (per serving of 12):***</u>

- Calories: 460
- Carbs: 31g
- Protein: 9g
- Fat: 28g
- Fiber: 10g
- Sugar: 19g

3.Cucumber Mint Popsicles

Revitalize your palate with Cucumber Mint Popsicles, a refreshing combination of crisp cucumber and lively mint. These popsicles provide a cool, hydrating treat that's perfect for scorching summer days. Every bite offers a burst of fresh flavor with a subtle sweetness, making them an excellent choice for a light, refreshing dessert. Crafted with genuine cucumber juice, fresh mint leaves, and a hint of honey, these popsicles are both nutritious and delectable. Savor the ultimate in cool relaxation with this invigorating frozen delight.

Cucumbers are mostly water and fiber, which helps with digestion. Their skin has fiber that helps food move through the digestive system faster. They are also high in B vitamins, which can help manage stress. Cucumbers have antioxidants and anti-inflammatory benefits that might help prevent cancer, boost brain health, lower heart disease risk, and aid in weight control. Unlike sugary or artificial treats, cucumbers are a healthier choice, offering hydration and important nutrients like vitamin K and potassium for strong bones and healthy blood pressure.

Preparation Time:
- Total Time:
- 4 hours 10 minutes (including freezing)

What You Need:
- 5 cups chopped cucumber (without seeds)
- ¾ cup fresh mint leaves
- ¾ cup lime juice
- ½ cup agave syrup
- ½ teaspoon sea salt

How to Make:
1. Blend the cucumber, mint, lime juice, agave syrup, and sea salt until smooth.
2. Pour the mix into 8 popsicle molds (4 ounces each).

3. Put popsicle sticks in.

4. Freeze for about 4 hours or until solid.

<u>*Nutrition (per pop):*</u>

- Calories: About 45
- Fat: 0 g
- Sodium: 30 mg
- Carbs: 12 g
- Sugars: 12 g
- Protein: 0 g

<u>*Tips:*</u>

- Add thin cucumber slices or whole mint leaves to each mold for extra flavor.
- Adjust agave syrup if you want a less sweet taste.
- To get popsicles out easily, run the outside of the molds under warm water briefly.

4. Coconut Macaroons

Coconut macaroons are sweet, chewy cookies made from shredded coconut, egg whites, and sugar. They have a crispy outside and a soft, moist inside, with a yummy coconut flavor. You can add chocolate or sea salt for extra taste. They're great for everyday eating or special events

Makes 26 macaroons

Preparation Time:

- 20 minutes
- Baking Time:
- 25 minutes
- Total Time:
- 45 minutes

ingredients:

- 1 bag (14 ounces) of sweetened shredded coconut (e.g., Baker's Angel Flake)
- ⅞ cup of sweetened condensed milk (see note for how to measure)
- 1 teaspoon of vanilla extract
- 2 large egg whites
- ¼ teaspoon of salt
- 4 ounces of good-quality semi-sweet chocolate, chopped (optional)

Instructions

1. Heat your oven to 325°F and set two racks in the middle. Put parchment paper on two baking sheets.

2. Mix shredded coconut, sweetened condensed milk, and vanilla extract in a bowl. In another bowl, beat egg whites and salt with a mixer until stiff. Gently mix the egg whites into the coconut mixture with a spatula.

3. Drop heaping tablespoons of the mixture onto the baking sheets, leaving about an inch between them. Bake for 23 to 25 minutes, switching the trays' positions halfway through, until they're golden. Let them cool on the trays for a few minutes, then move them to a wire rack to cool completely.

4. To add chocolate, melt it in a microwave-safe bowl, stirring every 30 seconds, or use a double boiler. Dip the bottoms of the cooled macaroons into the melted chocolate, let the excess drip off, and put them back on the baking sheets. Chill in the fridge for about 10 minutes to set the chocolate. Store in an airtight container at room temperature for up to a week.

- **<u>Note:</u>** The quality of coconut varies by brand. For best results, use Baker's Angel Flake (see the package in the first image on this page).

- **_Note:_** ⅞ cup equals ¾ cup plus 2 tablespoons.
- **_Note:_** Use parchment paper, not wax paper, on baking sheets. Wax paper makes macarons stick.

Freezer Tips: Macaroons can be frozen for up to 3 months. If you want to add chocolate, wait until they are thawed. Let macaroons cool completely, then store them in an airtight container with parchment paper or foil between layers. Let them warm to room temperature before serving.

Nutritional Info

Serving size:
- 1 macaroon (with optional chocolate)
- Calories:134, Fat: 8 g
- Saturated fat: 6 g, Carbs:16 g
- Sugar:15 g, Fiber:1 g, Protein:2 g
- Sodium: 81 mg, Cholesterol:4 mg

5. Sweet Potato Brownies

Sweet Potato Brownies are a tasty and healthier version of regular brownies. They are rich and fudgy because of the sweet potatoes, which make them naturally sweet and moist. The brownies are made by mixing cooked sweet potatoes into the batter, adding natural sweetness and extra nutrients. Ingredients like cocoa powder, almond flour, and vanilla are often used. These brownies are a delicious treat that's lower in sugar and full of vitamins, making them a great choice for a healthier dessert.

Vegan sweet potato brownies are perfect if you're looking for something low-calorie, gluten-free, or sugar-free. They also have a flourless option. Each brownie has 5.6 grams of protein and iron from cocoa, plus a vegetable serving. They mix great taste with good nutrition, making them a tasty yet healthy choice.

Preparetion Time:

- 20 minutes
- Bake Time:
- 20 minutes
- Total Time:
- 20 minutes
- Serves: 12 to 16 brownies

Ingredients:

- 3/4 cup sweet potato puree
- 1 cup peanut or almond butter (or another allergy-friendly butter)
- 1 tsp vanilla extract
- 6 tbsp flour (oat, white, spelt, or almond flour)
- 1/2 cup mini chocolate chips (plus more for the top, if you want)

- 2/3 cup sugar (use a sugar-free option for keto)
- 6 tbsp cocoa powder
- 1 1/2 tsp baking soda
- 1/8 tsp salt

Instructions:

1. Preheat your oven to 325°F. Line an 8-inch pan with parchment paper or grease it.

2. If your nut butter is hard, warm it a bit to soften.

3. Mix the nut butter with the sweet potato puree and vanilla extract until smooth.

4. In a separate bowl, mix the flour, chocolate chips, sugar, cocoa powder, baking soda, and salt.

5. Combine the dry mix with the wet mix and stir until you have a batter.

6. Pour the batter into the pan and smooth the top with another piece of parchment paper.

7. Bake for 20 minutes. The brownies will look soft and undercooked.

8. Let them cool to firm up. If they're too soft, chill them in the fridge for a few hours. Optionally, frost them if you like.

Per serving (1 brownie):

- Calories: 220
- Fat: 10g
- Saturated fat: 2g
- Cholesterol: 10mg
- Sodium: 50mg
- Total Carbohydrates: 30g
- Dietary Fiber: 4g
- Sugars: 20g
- Protein: 4g

Vitamins and Minerals:

- Vitamin A: 20% of the Daily Value (DV)
- Vitamin C: 10% of the DV
- Calcium: 4% of the DV
- Iron: 15% of the DV
- Potassium: 10% of the DV

<u>*Note*</u>

- The nutritional values may vary depending on the specific ingredients and portion sizes used.
- Sweet potatoes are a good source of fiber, vitamins, and minerals, making these brownies a slightly healthier option compared to traditional brownies.

6. Peach Crisp

Peach Crisp is a tasty dessert with soft peaches covered by a sweet and crunchy topping. The dessert is baked until the peaches are hot and the topping is golden and crisp. The topping is made with oats, brown sugar, butter, and a little cinnamon. It's often served warm with vanilla ice cream or whipped cream for extra flavor.

preparation time:

- 15minutes
- cooking time:
- 45 minutes
- Total time:1 hour
- makes 8 servings.

Ingredient

- For the peaches:
- 8 to 9 ripe peaches, pitted
- 1/4 cup brown sugar
- 2 tablespoons flour

- 1 teaspoon vanilla
- A small pinch of salt

For the topping:
- 1/2 cup melted butter
- 1/2 cup sugar
- 1/2 cup packed brown sugar
- 2/3 cup flour
- 2/3 cup oats
- 1/4 teaspoon salt

1. Heat your oven to 375°F. Butter a medium baking dish (an 11 x 7 oval dish is best, but a 9 x 9 square pan or 10-inch skillet will also work).

2. Remove the pits from the peaches and cut them into ¼-inch thick slices. Put the peach slices in the dish. Sprinkle With brown sugar, flour, and a bit of vanilla extract. Mix gently with your hands or a spoon, then spread the peaches out evenly.

3. For the topping, mix flour, oats, brown sugar, granulated sugar, salt, and butter in a bowl until it looks crumbly.

4. Spread the topping evenly over the peaches.

5. Bake for 40 to 45 minutes, until the peaches are bubbling and the topping is golden brown. Let it cool a little before serving. It tastes great with vanilla ice cream or whipped cream!

7.Apple Cinnamon Oat Bars

Apple Cinnamon Oat Bars are a tasty and healthy option for breakfast or a snack. Made with oats, apple pieces, and a touch of cinnamon, they're baked until golden and have a chewy texture with crispy edges. They're sweet and spicy, great for eating on the go and enjoying fall flavors anytime.

Preparetion Time:

- 10 minutes
- Cook Time:
- 25 minutes
- Total Time:
- 35 minutes
- Course: Breakfast, Dessert, Snack
- Servings: 9 squares

Ingredients

- 1 cup applesauce
- ⅓ cup almond butter
- 1 flax egg (1 tbsp ground flaxseed mixed with 2.5 tbsp water, let sit for 5 minutes)
- 2 tablespoons almond milk
- 1 teaspoon vanilla extract
- ¼ cup maple syrup
- 1 cup rolled oats
- 1 ¼ cups oat flour
- 1 teaspoon cinnamon
- 1 teaspoon baking powder
- 1 cup chopped apples

Instructions

1. Heat the oven to 350°F. Grease or line an 8x8 inch pan with parchment paper.

2. Make the flax egg by mixing 1 tbsp ground flaxseed with 2.5 tbsp water and letting it sit for 5 minutes.

3. In a bowl, mix oat flour, oats, cinnamon, and baking powder.

4. In another bowl, mix applesauce, almond butter, flax egg, almond milk, vanilla, and maple syrup.

5. Combine the dry ingredients with the wet ingredients and stir until mixed.

6. Fold in ⅔ cup of chopped apples.

7. Pour the mixture into the pan and top with the remaining chopped apples.

8. Bake for 25 minutes until the top is golden. Let cool in the pan for 10 minutes, then transfer to a rack to cool completely. Cut into bars and enjoy.

Per serving (1 bar):
- Calories: 250
- Fat: 8g
- Saturated fat: 1g
- Cholesterol: 0mg
- Sodium: 50mg
- Total Carbohydrates: 40g
- Dietary Fiber: 4g
- Sugars: 20g
- Protein: 3g

Vitamins and Minerals:

- Vitamin A: 2% of the Daily Value (DV)
- Vitamin C: 10% of the DV
- Calcium: 2% of the DV
- Iron: 10% of the DV
- Potassium: 8% of the DV

Additional nutrients:

- Antioxidants from apples and cinnamon
- Whole grain oats for added fiber and nutrition

Note:

- Nutritional values may vary depending on specific ingredients and portion sizes used.
- These bars are a good source of fiber, whole grains, and antioxidants, making them a healthier snack option.

8. Banana Bread

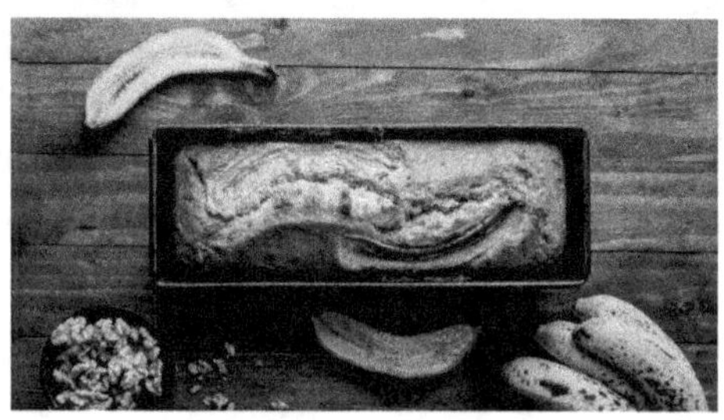

Banana bread is a soft, sweet cake made from ripe bananas, which makes it naturally sweet and fruity. It's usually made with basic ingredients like flour, sugar, eggs, and butter. You can add nuts, chocolate chips, or spices if you like. It's a dense and soft treat that's great for breakfast, a snack, or dessert. Banana bread is popular because it's easy to make and uses up old bananas.

Ingredients

- ½ cup unsalted butter, melted and slightly cooled
- ⅔ cup packed light brown sugar, soft and fresh
- 2 large eggs
- 3-4 ripe bananas, mashed (about 2 cups)
- 2 teaspoons vanilla extract
- 1 ¾ cups all-purpose flour*
- 1 teaspoon baking soda
- ¼ teaspoon salt
- ¼ cup brown sugar (for topping, optional)

Instructions

1. Heat your oven to 350°F.

2. In a large bowl, mix the melted butter with ⅔ cup brown sugar until combined, about 1 minute. Add eggs, bananas, and vanilla extract, and whisk until smooth.

3. In another bowl, mix the flour, baking soda, and salt. Fold this into the wet mixture with a spatula until just combined.

4. Grease a 9×9 inch pan, pour in the batter, and spread it out. Sprinkle the top with ¼ cup brown sugar if you like.

5. Bake for 20-25 minutes, turning the pan halfway. It's done when a toothpick inserted in the center comes out clean. Let cool on a wire rack.

Notes

- Flourb: Fluff the flour before measuring. You can mix 1 cup all-purpose flour with ¾ cup whole wheat flour if desired.
- Pan Options:
- Muffins: Bake in 12 muffin cups for about 15 minutes.
- 8×8 pan: Bake for 35-45 minutes.
- 9×5 loaf pan: Bake for 45-55 minutes.

Nutrition

- Calories: 212 kcal
- Carbs: 31g
- Protein: 3g
- Fat : 9g
- Saturated Fat : 5g
- Cholesterol : 51mg
- Sodium : 158 mg
- Potassium : 57mg
- Fiber : 1g
- Sugar : 16g

Nutritional values are estimates and may vary.

9. Maple Roasted Nuts

Maple Roasted Nuts are a tasty snack made by coating nuts like almonds, pecans, or walnuts with maple syrup and a little sea salt, then roasting them. This makes them sweet, salty, and crunchy. They're great to eat by themselves or to add on top of salads and desserts.

Preparation time:

- 10 minutes
- Total time:
- 10 minutes
- Makes:
- 8 portions

Ingredients

- 2 cups mixed nuts (like walnuts, pecans, almonds)
- 1/4 cup maple syrup
- 1/8 teaspoon salt
- 1 tablespoon sesame seeds (optional)

Instructions

1. Heat a dry pan over medium heat and toast the nuts for 3-5 minutes, stirring often.
2. Add the maple syrup and salt, and stir for another 3-5 minutes.
3. If you like, add sesame seeds before serving.

Tips & Notes

- Makes about 2 cups, or eight 1/4 cup servings.

Nutrition

- Calories: 247
- Carbs: 16 g
- Protein: 6 g
- Fat: 19 g
- Saturated Fat: 3 g
- Sodium: 42 mg
- Potassium: 242 mg
- Fiber: 3 g
- Sugar: 6 g

- Vitamin C: 1 mg
- Calcium: 46 mg
- Iron: 1 mg

10. Fig and Date Energy Balls

Fig and Date Energy Balls are small, healthy snacks made from dried figs, dates, and nuts. They're sweet, high in fiber, and full of vitamins and minerals. These snacks are great for a quick boost of energy and make a tasty, healthy choice instead of processed snacks.

Preparation Time:

- 15 minutes
- Total Time:
- 15 minutes
- Makes about 18 bite-sized pieces

Ingredients

- 15 dried Mission figs (about 6 oz)
- 7 pitted Medjool dates (around 4 oz)
- ¼ cup natural almond butter
- ¾ cup old-fashioned rolled oats (use quick-cooking oats or gluten-free if needed)
- ¼ cup ground flaxseed meal
- 1 teaspoon vanilla extract

Instructions

1. Put all ingredients into a large food processor.

2. Pulse a few times to mix, then scrape down the sides with a spatula.

3. Blend for 2-3 minutes until the mixture forms clumps and sticks to the bowl. Scrape down the sides as needed.

4. Roll the mixture into balls of any size you like. Store in an airtight container in the fridge for up to two weeks.

Extra Tips

- Storage: Keep these energy balls in the fridge for up to 14 days. They're good straight from the fridge but taste better if left out for a few minutes.

- Freezing: You can freeze the energy balls for up to 3 months. Just thaw them in the fridge overnight before eating.

- Calories: 89
- Carbohydrates: 15 g
- Protein: 2 g
- Fat: 3 g
- Saturated Fat: 1 g
- Polyunsaturated Fat: 1 g
- Monounsaturated Fat: 1 g
- Potassium: 167 mg
- Fiber: 3 g
- Sugar: 10 g
- Vitamin A: 15 IU
- Vitamin C: 1 mg
- Calcium: 36 mg
- Iron: 1 mg

These energy bites are a convenient snack, offering natural sugars, healthy fats, and fiber. They're perfect for a quick energy boost or a pre/post-workout snack.

Extra Bonus: 30-Day Vegan Meal Prep Plan for Vestibular Migraine Relief

The "30-Day Vegan Meal Prep Plan for Vestibular Migraine Relief" is a guide to help people manage vestibular migraines with a vegan diet. It includes simple, nutritious recipes for breakfast, lunch, dinner, and snacks that avoid common migraine triggers. The meals are packed with anti-inflammatory foods like leafy greens, nuts, seeds, and whole grains, and avoid things like caffeine, processed foods, and high-histamine items. The plan also gives tips on how to prepare meals efficiently, keep things varied, and track how different foods affect you. This plan aims to improve overall health and reduce the number and intensity of vestibular migraines.

Day 1

- **Breakfast:** Vegan Banana Pancakes
- **Lunch:** Sweet Potato and Black Beans Tacos
- **Dinner:** Sweet Potato Stew

Day 2

- **Breakfast:** Vegan Blueberry Muffins
- **Lunch:** Stuffed Cherry Tomatoes
- **Dinner:** Butternut Squash Soup

Day 3

- **Breakfast:** Millet Porridge
- **Lunch:** Avocado Toast
- **Dinner:** Fingerling Potato Salad

Day 4

Breakfast: Vegan Breakfast Cookies

Lunch: Roasted Red Pepper Hummus with Raw Carrots

Dinner: Boursin Stuffed Mushrooms

Day 5

- **Breakfast:** Vegan Banana Bread Waffles
- **Lunch:** Peach Burrata Salad
- **Dinner:** Sweet Potato and Black Beans

Day 6

- **Breakfast:** Coconut Yogurt Parfait
- **Lunch:** Caesar Salad Dressing without Anchovies with Butter Lettuce Salad
- **Dinner:** Flavorful Buddha Bowl

Day 7

- **Breakfast:** Vegan Breakfast Burritos
- **Lunch:** Crispy Chickpeas Snack with a side salad

- **_Dinner:_** Mozzarella Alfredo Pasta Sauce with Veggies

Day 8

- **_Breakfast:_** Vegan Banana Bread
- **_Lunch:_** Quinoa Porridge with fresh fruits
- **_Dinner:_** Sweet Potato Stew

Day 9

- **_Breakfast:_** Vegan Blueberry Muffins
- **_Lunch:_** Stuffed Cherry Tomatoes
- **_Dinner:_** Butternut Squash Soup

Day 10

- **_Breakfast:_** Avocado Toast
- **_Lunch:_** Roasted Red Pepper Hummus with Raw Carrots
- **_Dinner:_** Fingerling Potato Salad

Day 11

- **Breakfast:** Vegan Breakfast Cookies
- **Lunch:** Peach Burrata Salad
- **Dinner:** Boursin Stuffed Mushrooms

Day 12

- **Breakfast:** Vegan Banana Pancakes
- **Lunch:** Sweet Potato and Black Beans Tacos
- **Dinner:** Sweet Potato and Black Beans

Day 13

- **Breakfast:** Millet Porridge
- **Lunch:** Coconut Yogurt Parfait
- **Dinner:** Flavorful Buddha Bowl

Day 14

- **Breakfast:** Vegan Banana Bread Waffles

- **Lunch:** Caesar Salad Dressing without Anchovies with Butter Lettuce Salad
- **Dinner:** Mozzarella Alfredo Pasta Sauce with Veggies

Day 15

- **Breakfast:** Vegan Breakfast Burritos
- **Lunch:** Crispy Chickpeas Snack
- **Dinner:** Sweet Potato Stew

Day 16

- **Breakfast:** Vegan Blueberry Muffins
- **Lunch:** Stuffed Cherry Tomatoes
- **Dinner:** Butternut Squash Soup

Day 17

- **Breakfast:** Coconut Yogurt Parfait
- **Lunch:** Quinoa Porridge with fresh fruits
- **Dinner:** Fingerling Potato Salad

Day 18

- ***Breakfast:*** Vegan Breakfast Cookies
- ***Lunch:*** Roasted Red Pepper Hummus with Raw Carrots
- ***Dinner:*** Boursin Stuffed Mushrooms

Day 19

- ***Breakfast:*** Vegan Banana Pancakes
- ***Lunch:*** Peach Burrata Salad
- ***Dinner:*** Sweet Potato and Black Beans

Day 20

- ***Breakfast:*** Vegan Banana Bread
- ***Lunch:*** Flavorful Buddha Bowl
- ***Dinner:*** Mozzarella Alfredo Pasta Sauce with Veggies

Day 21

- **Breakfast:** Vegan Blueberry Muffins
- **Lunch:** Sweet Potato and Black Beans Tacos
- **Dinner:** Sweet Potato Stew

Day 22

- **Breakfast:** Millet Porridge
- **Lunch:** Stuffed Cherry Tomatoes
- **Dinner:** Butternut Squash Soup

Day 23

- **Breakfast:** Vegan Breakfast Cookies
- **Lunch:** Roasted Red Pepper Hummus with Raw Carrots
- **Dinner:** Fingerling Potato Salad

Day 24

- **Breakfast:** Vegan Banana Pancakes

- **_Lunch:_** Peach Burrata Salad
- **_Dinner:_** Boursin Stuffed Mushrooms

Day 25

- **_Breakfast:_** Coconut Yogurt Parfait
- **_Lunch:_** Vegan Breakfast Burritos
- **_Dinner:_** Mozzarella Alfredo Pasta Sauce with Veggies

Day 26

- **_Breakfast:_** Vegan Banana Bread Waffles
- **_Lunch:_** Caesar Salad Dressing without Anchovies with Butter Lettuce Salad
- **_Dinner:_** Sweet Potato and Black Beans

Day 27

- **_Breakfast:_** Vegan Blueberry Muffins
- **_Lunch:_** Crispy Chickpeas Snack
- **_Dinner:_** Sweet Potato Stew

Day 28

- **_Breakfast:_** Millet Porridge
- **_Lunch:_** Coconut Yogurt Parfait
- **_Dinner:_** Flavorful Buddha Bowl

Day 29

- **_Breakfast:_** Vegan Breakfast Cookies
- **_Lunch:_** Stuffed Cherry Tomatoes
- **_Dinner:_** Butternut Squash Soup

Day 30

- **_Breakfast:_** Vegan Banana Pancakes
- **_Lunch:_** Peach Burrata Salad
- **_Dinner:_** Mozzarella Alfredo Pasta Sauce with Veggies

This plan incorporates a range of recipes to keep your meals exciting while adhering to a vegan diet that's suitable for managing vestibular migraines. Adjust portions and snacks based on your personal preferences and nutritional needs.

<u>Conclusion</u>

In conclusion, the "Vegan Diet Cookbook for Vestibular Migraine" by Anita F. McCluskey is a valuable guide for those dealing with vestibular migraines and following a vegan diet. This cookbook offers a range of tasty recipes that are specifically designed to help manage migraines while sticking to a vegan lifestyle.

Inside, you'll find easy-to-follow recipes along with helpful tips on how to avoid migraine triggers and improve your overall health. By using these recipes every day, you're taking an important step towards feeling better.

The book also provides advice on meal planning and making healthy food choices, making it easier for you to stick to a diet that supports your well-being. It's not just about cooking; it's about making smarter health decisions.

By following the advice and recipes in this book, you're investing in your health and working towards managing your migraines more effectively. We hope this cookbook helps you feel better and brings positive changes to your life.

We wish you all the best on your journey to improved health and happiness. May each day bring you closer to feeling great.